A BEHAVIORAL VISION APPROACH FOR PERSONS WITH PHYSICAL DISABILITIES

BY WILLIAM V. PADULA, O.D.

OPTOMETRIC EXTENSION PROGRAM

Copyright © 1988

All rights reserved. No part of this work covered by the copyright herein may be reproduced or used in any form or by any means—graphic, electronic, or mechanical, including photocopying, recording, taping, or information storage and retrieval systems—without permission of the publisher.

Printed in the United States of America

Published by Optometric Extension Program Foundation, Inc.
2912 South Daimler Street
Santa Ana, CA 92705-5811

Managing Editor: Sally Marshall Corngold

First Edition, 1988
Library of Congress Cataloging in Publication Data
Padula, William V.
    A behavioral vision approach for persons with physical disabilities/ by William V. Padula.
        p.   cm.
    Bibliography: p.
    ISBN 0-943599-04-0 : $49.50
    1. Behavioral optometry. 2. Vision disorders--Patients--Rehabilitation. I. Title.
    [DNLM: 1. Behavior. 2. Vision Disorders--rehabilitation. 3. Visual Perception. WW 140 P125b]
    RE960.P33 1988
    617.7--dc19
    DNLM/DLC
    for Library of Congress   88-37450
                                                          CIP

DEDICATION

To Judie, Bill, and Lauren for their love, patience, and support.

ABOUT THE AUTHORS

(In order of appearance in text)

William V. Padula, O.D., F.A.A.O.

William V. Padula, O.D., is a graduate of Pennsylvania College of Optometry and is a Fellow of the American Academy of Optometry. He serves as Director of the Low Vision Clinic at the Rehabilitation Center in New Haven, Ct., and was the Founding Chairman of the Low Vision Section for the American Optometric Association. He has served as National Consultant in Low Vision Services for the American Foundation for the Blind and Consultant to the National Institute of Human Development. He has consulted and developed a low vision clinic named in his honor at the Zhongshan Eye Research Hospital in Canton, China and regularly consults with the Centro de Aprendizaje de Cuernavaca, Mexico. He is on staff at the New Britain Memorial Hospital, consults with many programs for head-injured persons throughout the United States and is a State Police Surgeon with the Connecticut State Police.

Dr. Padula has written numerous publications and is in private practice in Guilford, Connecticut.

Jannie Shapiro, M.Ed.

Jannie Shapiro is Coordinator of the Low Vision Clinic at the Rehabilitation Center, New Haven, Connecticut. Her responsibilities include providing functional vision screenings for multi-handicapped children and adults with strokes and traumatic brain injuries; evaluation of a patient's gait, coordination, and movement abilities; and training in the use of dispensed low vision aids for near and distance viewing. Prior to her working at the Low Vision Clinic, Mrs. Shapiro was an orientation and mobility specialist at Oak Hill School in Hartford, Connecticut, where she instituted a functional vision evaluation program for the school's multihandicapped population.

Christine A. Nelson, Ph.D., O.T.R., F.A.O.T.A.

Christine A. Nelson earned her M.S. in Child Development from the University of Wisconsin and completed certification in Neurodevelopmental (Bobath) Treatment in 1963. Dr. Nelson was certified as an NDT Coordinator-Instructor by Dr. and Mrs. Karel Bobath in 1973 after completing requirements for her Ph.D. in Human Development at the University of Maryland.

Dr. Nelson began her career in occupational therapy, working with physically disabled and blind children, moving from institutional to community to private settings. Her direct treatment of multihandicapped children, her experience in developmental assessment and her preparation of therapists to work with children with neuromotor disorders have prepared her to share these practical insights into problems of posture and movement as they relate to visual impairment. She has authored a chapter on Cerebral Palsy in "Neurological Rehabilitation" by Mosby, has participated in the making of two films and has written several other chapters and articles recently. She is now Clinical Coordinator of the Centro de Aprendizaje de Cuernavaca, Mexico.

Laurel L. Watson, M.A.

Laurel L. Watson received her B.S. from Northern Illinois University and her M.A. from San Francisco State University. Her experiences in public schools has afforded her opportunities to continue learning from teachers, therapists, optometrists and students.

She coordinates citywide programs for children with visual impairments for Chicago Public Schools.

Kathleen M. Newman, M.A.

Kathleen M. Newman received her M.A. from the University of Northern Colorado as a teacher of the visually impaired and an orientation and mobility specialist. With 15 years of experience in movement and visual impairment, she has come to believe that maximum student potential can best be achieved by incorporating the bases of visual and motor learning into functional activities.

She has participated in organizing vision programs in several states and is currently employed in Nebraska by Lincoln Public Schools.

Gwen K. Neitzel, R.P.T.

Gwen K. Neitzel received her pediatric physical therapy training at Northwestern University Medical School. A former elementary school teacher, she is currently employed at Luther Hospital in Eau Claire, Wisconsin, where she developed, and now manages, a comprehensive industrial rehabilitation program while continuing to serve as a pediatric therapy consultant.

Judith A. Padula

Judith A. Padula graduated from Dominican College in Blauvelt, New York and has been a teacher in Connecticut for over 10 years, working with visually impaired and multihandicapped children. She has co-authored publications about low vision rehabilitation for visually impaired children and the affect on academic performance. She has coordinated visual stimulation and vision therapy programs for low vision children in the school system and optometric private practices.

W. Michael Magrun, M.S.

W. Michael Magrun received his Masters of Science in Occupational Therapy from the State University of New York at Buffalo in 1974. For the past 15 years he has specialized in the treatment of children with neuro-motor disorders and learning disabilities. He is a former instructor of pediatric occupational therapy at the SUNY at New York and the University of Central Arkansas. He holds certification in neuro-developmental treatment for children and babies. His practice has centered around the understanding, evaluation and treatment of movement and postural disorganization and disability as it relates to developmental disorders and learning. Mr. Magrun has published articles on the subject in the American Journal of Occupational Therapy, Somatics Journal, Occupational Therapy in Health Care and the Arkansas Occupational Therapy Association News-Journal. Currently, Magrun is in private practice as a consultant.

ACKNOWLEDGMENT

This book is the product of years spent working with patients with many types of disabilities. I wish to thank each patient for sharing his unique experiences and problems with me. I also wish to thank the following professionals whose discussions and writings enabled me to develop the concepts presented in this book: R. Apell, O.D., C. Forkiotos, O.D., A. Shankman, O.D., C. Nelson, O.D., J. Streff, O.D., and the late A. Gesell, M.D.

TABLE OF CONTENTS

	page
Dedication	iii
About the Authors	iv
Acknowledgement	viii
List of Photos	xi
List of Figures	xii
List of Tables	xii
Preface	xiii

Chapter I.   Vision: The Process - William V. Padula, O.D.   1

Chapter II.   Development of the Visually Impaired Child - William V. Padula, O.D.   12

Chapter III.   Perceptual Development of the Sighted Child - William V. Padula, O.D.   18

Chapter IV.   Perceptual Development of the Visually Impaired Child - William V. Padula, O.D.   30

Chapter V.   Defining the Impairment and Developing a Model of Services - William V. Padula, O.D., and Jannie Shapiro, M.Ed.   41

Chapter VI.   Postural Development and Vision - Christine Nelson, Ph.D., O.T.R.   46

Chapter VII.   Visual-Perceptual Developmental Needs of the Visually Impaired Child - William V. Padula, O.D.   55

Chapter VIII.   Low-Vision Service Delivery System and Its Future - William V. Padula, O.D.   82

Chapter IX.	Enhancing Vision and Motor Skills in the Learning Environment - Laurel L. Watson, M.A., Kathleen M. Newman, M.A. and Gwen K. Neitzel, R.P.T.	92
Chapter X.	Low Vision and Education for the School-Age Child - William V. Padula, O.D. and Judith A. Padula	103
Chapter XI.	The Multihandicapped Child - William V. Padula, O.D.	123
Chapter XII.	Positioning Aspects of Successful Visual Intervention - Christine Nelson, Ph.D., O.T.R	134
Chapter XIII.	Evaluating Quality in Motor Behavior - W. Michael Magrun, M.S.	152
Chapter XIV.	Post-trauma Vision Syndrome Caused by Head Injury - William V. Padula, O.D. and Jannie Shapiro, M.Ed.	167
Bibliography		187

LIST OF PHOTOS

		page
A.	Vision and posture	47
B.	Prone without extension	47
C.	Pivot prone	48
D.	Baby extension	48
E.	Baby flexion	48
F.	Infant stabilizing to direct gaze	49
G.	Protective extension	52
H.	Movement on floor	53
I.	Normal posture	135
J.	Abnormal posture	135
K.	Sitting between legs	136
L.	Poor control and high tone	136
M.	Normal fixing to focus	138
N.	High tone moving	138
O.	Abnormal posture with visual focus	140
P.	Sitting with symmetry	141
Q.	Skilled movement	143
R.	Severely involved child--multihandicapped	144
S.	Active treatment	145
T.	Therapy	145
U.	Baby with low tonus	147
V.	Positioning in sitting	150
W.	Positioning	150

LIST OF FIGURES

                                                                                    page

1. Child development demonstrated as a relationship between physical, psychological, and environmental variables. 31

2. Abnormal child development demonstrated by variations in support between physical, psychological, and environmental variables. 31

3. Presentation of a Classroom Program 101

4. Graph: Normal and Abnormal Tonus 146

5. Post-Trauma Vision Syndrome 171

LIST OF TABLES

1. Development of the Normally-Sighted Child 20

2. Development of the Blind Child 33

PREFACE

A number of years ago, when I was an optometry student, a professor told our class that we must develop our own model of vision and practice optometry according to the philosophy that fits that model. I remember afterwards how puzzled we all were over our professor's words. What did he mean, "A model of vision?" It seemed perfectly clear, after four years of studying optometry, there was only one model of vision: The eye optically focuses light onto the retina, and in turn the light is converted into chemical and electrical signals that traverse via the optic nerve to the cortex where sight occurs.

The eye is an extremely complex organ that can be diagnosed of pathology or malfunction. We have gained greater understanding of the complexity of the eye with the advent of new technology that can analyze ocular pressure, retinal integrity, oculomotor function, image transmission to the cortex, and contrast sensitivity, as well as to quantify information about the eye and the transfer of signals to the brain. Through mathematical constructs and the advancement of physiological optics, reaction time, muscle function, color perception, nerve transmission, and many other ocular functions can be differentiated and analyzed. Binocularity also can be quantified, and muscle balance problems, suppressions and anomalous retinal fixation sites dealt with by structured therapeutic programs designed to change the function of the eyes.

At the time, this model seemed complete. If a problem could not be analyzed through either observable details or quantified through other diagnostic procedures, then the symptoms were of psychosomatic origin. This line of demarcation was clear cut. Psychosomatic problems were supposedly not visual and belonged in the realm of other professionals.

While practicing optometry, however, I encountered patients who did not seem to fit this model. Initially, I remember discounting patients' symptoms or thinking to myself that they were psychological. Over time, many of these patients caused me to question the model that I practiced. Why did the child with 20/400 acuity and no ocular or cortical pathology, and who reported seeing objects float around the room, suddenly improve to 20/40 with stable vision when an empty eyeglass frame was placed before his eyes? Why did the 65-year-old woman with cataracts, who had no balance or mobility problems with 20/200 acuity, suddenly have to walk down the hall holding the walls after her cataracts were removed and her acuity was 20/20? Why did the multihandicapped child align his deviated eye after his therapist changed his neck and shoulder posture? Why did a person develop problems with walking and balance and begin to neglect her right side after a cerebralvascular accident that caused a right-field loss but no impairment to motor function? Why did two seven-year-old, visually impaired children of similar intelligence, each with Stargardt's macular degeneration and 20/200 acuity, function so differently? One showed significant developmental delays and problems with motor organization and balance, while the other was scoring in the top 10 percent of her class and was involved with a variety of sports and other activities. These are only a few examples of patients whose symptoms did not fit my model.

As the whys accumulated, it became apparent that something was missing from this model of vision. To account for these variations in performance, I decided that the psychology of vision somehow must play an important role in our function and performance. So, with this premise, I redesigned and expanded my model of vision. Through my study of child development, movement, posture, reflexes, motor function (normal and abnormal, impaired and unimpaired), it became apparent that the process of vision was much more involved. I found it was more closely related to perception, balance, movement, development, sensory and motor organization and cognitive function than I had originally believed.

In my search for a means to evaluate the dynamic process of vision in relationship to these variables, it became increasingly difficult to quantify the information according to traditional approaches of optometry. Therefore, behavior was observed in an attempt to both understand the psychology of vision and to develop treatment approaches that deal with the blend of the physiology of vision as well as its psychology.

There is need to use behavioral approaches in vision care with patients who have sensory and motor impairments. This book is intended to cause the reader to ask questions about his or her own model and mode of practice, whether it be in optometry, ophthalmology, therapy or education. While the authors have been and are presently involved in research concerning the approaches discussed herein, the purpose of this text is to provide a framework for further study and practice of behavioral vision care for persons affected by sensory and motor impairments. This book provides an overview of information about development, vision impairment, neuro-motor function, multi-handicapped, and traumatic brain-injured persons.

This book provides an overview of information about development, vision impairment, neuro-motor function, and multi-handicapped and traumatic brain injured persons.

CHAPTER I

VISION: THE PROCESS

Vision is a behavior that in many instances is predictable. However, one must not assume that vision will develop on a rigid time table or that all children or adults will demonstrate similar behaviors at a particular stage. Fortunately, people are too dynamic to allow development to proceed in a totally predictable manner. Certain stages of development can be identified nevertheless by averaging the development of many children.

It is important to understand that the child attempts to organize sensory and motor processes through the use of the dynamic process of vision. The child unconsciously incorporates aspects of previous development and sensory-motor function as experience. He utilizes experience as a means to manipulate and reinterpret new information, thereby establishing a developmental sequence of knowledge. This process is ongoing and continuous throughout a person's life. It must also be recognized that experience can become a means of distorting reality. What we have seen or felt or experienced influences our interpretation of future events.

It can be assumed, through analysis of the neurology of sensory-motor processes within the body, that vision plays a primary role in learning. There are over 1,900,000 nerve fibers that exit each eye. These represent approximately 70 percent of the sensory nerve fibers in the entire body. Therefore, a major amount of information is received by the cortex through the eyeballs each second.

Concerning developmental anatomy, the eyeballs are a direct extension of the brain, or cortex. During fetal development optic vesicles extend forward from the visual cortex to align in the anterior segments of the cranium. The optic vesicles become the eyeballs. The extension arm of the optic vesicles later becomes the optic nerve and optic track, which deliver messages from the eyeball to the visual cortex located in the posterior portion of the brain.

Nerve fibers emanating from the macula, or the central areas of the eyes, will align centrally in the optic nerve and optic track and localize themselves in central areas in the visual cortex. Peripheral fibers from the eyes orient themselves in the optic nerve and optic track around the central fibers and align themselves in peripheral areas of the visual cortex.

The imaging of our visual world occupies a major portion of our attention and cognition. Most people take vision for granted; a sensory function that delivers information to the brain, much like a computer. In some ways the high organization of the visual system which leads to visual imagery has lead to our own restrictions and limitations in understanding how the visual process works. Because we are highly involved in cognitive function, we have limited awareness of the systems related to movement, posture, and in general the motor system.

Our individual sensory processors (eyes, ears, nose, tongue, mouth and fingers) lead us to interpret our own organization as isolated systems. This isolation has brought about the establishment of highly specialized professions such as optometry, ophthalmology, and audiology, as well as specialists in olfaction. While this approach is effective in providing treatment for a specific sensory organ, it is not effective in dealing with problems relating to a combination of sensory-motor functions. Problems involving sensory-motor coordination have been termed by some as integration problems. However, all sensory and motor processes are already integrated neurologically unless there is physical deformity. When a person attempts to combine sensory and motor function but has difficulty, one should not assume that the difficulty is an integration problem. The difficulty might actually stem from an inability to discern differences in sensory-motor function (Streff, 1976) and in utilizing information from the sensory and motor processes as feedback to organize performance. Understanding this, a rehabilitative effort should be thought of in terms of how the individual discerns differences between motor and sensory information.

The integration of the neurological system in the cortex requires that information be shared and matched between sensory and motor processes. For example, some individuals have stated that when they take their glasses off they have a difficult time hearing. It may be understood that the visual process of these individuals needs to match information with the hearing process. Another notable example illustrates how balance is affected. It can be observed that when standing on one foot, balance is diminished for many individuals when their eyes are closed. The interpretation might be that the visual process is sharing and matching information with other components such as the vestibular system and the kinesthetic process, both of which are important to balance and movement.

In an attempt to understand behaviors, we must try to think of them as a representation of the way in which the person both interprets information and organizes information through all of the sensory-motor processes. This point will become clearer as discussion of the performance of individuals with motor or sensory impairments is developed.

With this as background, we can now attempt to understand vision as it relates to behavior and then develop a model which will provide us with a basis for rehabilitation. Researchers such as Liebowitz, Post and Trevarethan have received greater acclaim in psychology than they have in the field of vision care. The reason might be that it is easier to understand the research than it is to make that information practical to the clinician.

In a general manner, let's consider what the visual process is, according to these researchers, and attempt to develop a basis for a behavioral and clinical model. The visual system is composed of not one but two components: a central, or focal, process and a peripheral, or ambient, process. Neurologically, as we discussed earlier, the central process is delivered primarily through the macula, which is located on the retina at the central or posterior pole of the eye. The macula is composed of cone cells which deliver the highest resolution, or visual acuity. Nerve fibers from this area exit the eye through the optic nerve and emanate to central areas of the visual cortex. A primary function of cone cells is color detection. The peripheral area of the retina is mainly composed of rods. The farther away from the macula, the fewer observable cones there are in the retina. The rod cells are predominant in this peripheral area and are more important to scotopic vision, or lower-threshold luminosity. Nerve fibers delivered from peripheral areas of the retina extend through the optic nerve and tract to more peripheral areas of the cortex.

Although, as mentioned earlier, we are concerned with the visual image delivered primarily from central vision function, it must be noted that neurologically many nerve cells delivered from the eye do not reach highly organized seeing areas in the cortex. These fibers from more peripheral areas of the retina will drop off without reaching areas related to seeing visual images. Many of the fibers drop off to link up in the mid-brain with other areas that relate to motor and sensory functions. The focal process of vision is attention-oriented and is delivered primarily through macula and paramacula areas of the retina, thus allowing us to center in on detail.

The peripheral process is ambient in function and expansive and is more involved with spatial orientation and awareness than detail detection. Noting the neuroanatomy of the eyes and brain, the ambient process of vision relates very importantly to the motor system. The detail or focal process is a fairly recent development in the millions of years that it has taken our visual process to organize and evolve. The frog, for example, has a visual process that is spatially oriented. It is designed to detect movement for the purpose of food detection and survival against predators. An experiment demonstrated that a frog placed in a box was unable to detect a dead fly hanging from the ceiling, and within a week starved to death. In a similar experiment, a frog did not detect the dead fly for several days, but when a live fly was placed in the box, the movement of the fly was immediately detected and the frog caught it.

Primates have a high level of visual function combined with the focal process. Humans have the highest level of all. The focal process of vision develops with maturity and enables the person to center in on detail. Analyzing the relationship of the focal and ambient processes to human neurological development, we discover that nerve fibers from the central macula are not myelinated at birth. The signals received from the macular area are not as distinct at birth as they are weeks later. For this reason the visual process of the newborn is highly spatially oriented. This ambient spatial process of vision is designed for several reasons. It seems that a newborn infant's primary purpose is to organize his motor function, to gain control of limbs, head movements, etc. As we discussed, many of the nerve fibers of the eye are not delivered to higher cortical levels involving areas of imaging or seeing, but are oriented in mid-brain or lower brain stem, linking up with motor centers for balance, movement, and coordination. Developmentally, the lack of focal vision process enables the young infant to orient the ambient process of vision and reinforce efforts to organize motor control.

As motor function becomes organized, the focal process of vision develops in an attempt to refine motor function. These motor experiences later provide a base for higher level sensory discrimination. The ability to match information between the senses and the motor processes yields coordination of motor function. The limitations of one sense or motor process will alter the experience and affect how information can be matched. A limitation to the visual process will alter the effects on the motor system and vice versa. The matching of information between these processes should be fluid at infancy. As the child develops, he will begin to organize movement of a limb, such as the arm and hand, and at about the same time the child will begin to fixate a more focal component of the visual process on the hand. This interchange between the focal and the ambient function of vision continues throughout the child's development.

The process of vision is established through the motor system. Through the motor system the sensory system functions. There is an intrinsic value established by the extraocular-motor system and its relationship to the kinesthetic and vestibular systems. The kinesthetic and vestibular systems are very important in developing ocular-motor control.

Rudimentary experiences involving eye movements in relation to posture and gravity actually begin during fetal development. Postural adjustments of the fetus that occur as righting responses to gravity and to the spatial environment, primarily initiated through vestibular and kinesthetic interaction, have been monitored when the expectant mother shifts her body. These reflexes initiate rudimentary movements of the eyes through the ocular muscles in late stages of fetal development. It is the motor component of vision that develops first and provides information about spatial position. This information is continually matched with information from kinesthetic and proprioceptive systems. It is the motor component of vision that provides a base for sensory function.

Researchers have found that the sensory function of vision ceases when the motor component of vision, namely, the extraocular muscles, is paralyzed. There are minor flicks and tremors of the ocular muscles that cause the eyes to be in constant motion. These flicks and tremors never permit the image of the environment to remain stable on the retina. When the eye muscles are paralyzed with a drug such as curare that stops these flicks and tremors, sensory imagery ceases. It is not until the effects of the drug wear off that seeing, or imaging, reoccurs.

In addition, spatial constructs of the visual environment are affected by the ocular-motor relationship. It has been reported that when there is a tendency for the eyes to diverge (exophoria), there is a flattening effect on depth perception; a convergence tendency (esophoria) does not. Esophoria and exophoria are states of ocular-motor balance. Some believe that these states are simply muscle imbalances. However, if one attempts to understand the dynamic interchange between motor processing and sensory processing of vision throughout the child's development, additional questions of what the states of exophoria and esophoria really indicate must be asked. These states may indicate relationships between sensory-motor involvement. Amounts of esophoria and exophoria will vary during different developmental stages, and correlations between these ocular-motor states and the stages of development do exist. The purpose of this discussion is to establish a model for thinking that will provide a behavioral approach to rehabilitation which can be used through the visual process. This approach will go far beyond a sensory model.

The style of vision continues throughout life. The patterns established by the way a person utilizes the focal and ambient functions of vision are reinforced through motor relationships. The perceptual aspects of vision are very much influenced by the motor functions of this process. This creates a dynamic interchange that is quite different from sensory models that are often used to describe sight. Sight, therefore, is a static concept of seeing that does not necessarily equate performance and motor function.

The model of vision which we have now developed can be applied to developmental performance and behavior. This model will provide us with new insights into posture and movement, which are primary when considering either the development of a child or of multihandicapped and traumatic brain-injured individuals. In the following chapters we will attempt to understand the visual process and how to create environments for change.

Time, Space and Movement

The development of concepts of spatial parameters and timing are very important to the overall development of the child. Depth perception has been studied by researchers for many years. Classical experiments have indicated that certain factors of depth perception are innate. In one experiment, a kitten was placed on a table that was painted in black and white checkerboard patterns. The table also had a cliff that was covered with clear Plexiglas. The kitten demonstrated caution when it approached the cliff and refused to walk onto the Plexiglas, suggesting that for this two-eyed animal there was an understanding of depth perception and that caution was demonstrated because the kitten saw the cliff.

In another classical experiment done by Richard Held, Ph.D., a kitten was placed in a carousel that was attached to a harness. A second kitten was attached to the harness. The kitten in the carousel was denied motor movement from birth. The kitten that pulled the carousel had been permitted the opportunity to move. Both kittens were binocular. The results of this experiment were that the first kitten, after being taken from the carousel, did not have accurate depth perception, balance or motor movement, whereas the second kitten had a much greater ability to judge depth. This research experiment demonstrates that the visual process establishes order of depth perception through the structure and reinforcement of the motor system.

We must ask ourselves, what are we testing for in a visual examination that requires that the child or person remain stationary in a chair to read visual acuity charts and have a refraction performed? Also, what is really determined by depth perception tests that do not permit motor interaction or object localization? It has been stated in literature that individuals with strabismus (an eye malalignment) who also demonstrate suppression (a lack of binocularity) have little or no depth perception when tested. However, it has been the author's experience that when individuals with zero percent depth perception, as measured on stereopsis tests, are permitted to reach up and touch a pencil, their depth perception is considerably reduced when the strabismic eye is covered. Why, then, does this individual with no depth perception on a stereopsis test and with suppression of one eye have difficulty localizing objects in space when the strabismic eye is covered? It is possible that such tests examine only one aspect of binocularity and depth perception. Further, it is likely that individuals, even with high angle strabismus turns of the eye, can still utilize aspects of ambient visual processing in the strabismic eye to match enough information to have improved depth perception when using both eyes.

Present forms of visual testing permit limited interaction of motor and visual functions. Unless the visual process is examined as a dynamic process involving kinesthetic and proprioceptive reinforcement, findings from the examination will be limited, leading to possible misinterpretation. Ideally, the visual examination for individuals with sensory and/or motor handicaps should include both perceptual-motor evaluation and a detailed vision examination, enabling the clinician to behaviorally observe the individual in an attempt to understand gross and fine motor abilities in relationship to visual function.

Since movement is a critical component to the development of spatial-visual relationships, movement must also be related to the development of time relationships. Time and space experiences develop through an interchange of sensory and motor function. What does distance mean to the newborn infant who looks across the room without having had the opportunity to move on all fours? It is through his motor system that the child first understands space by crawling across the floor to develop interaction between motor, visual and other sensory processes. The child may see but does not have a meaningful experience until he is able to crawl or move. The kitten experiment demonstrates that depth is an innate observation; however, accurate object localization must be refined through sensory-motor interaction. This experience, once established, can be matched to new visual experiences, allowing the child an understanding of depth perception even in new environmental surroundings.

Rudimentary time relationships are established at very early ages. Even in fetal development, the child experiences the rhythm of his own heart, the beating of his mother's heart and the rhythm of respiration. These rhythms are experienced early in fetal development through somato-sensory stimulation and later with the development of the auditory system. These rudimentary concepts of timing continue after the child is born and further develop as a spatial reference when movement is established. As the child moves through space, time is represented by how long it takes him to go from one point to the next. Once established, this information enables the child to match it with new auditory and/or visual information so he can judge how long it will take to move from one point to another. This process uses higher level sensory processing. However, it must be emphasized that the basis of this interpretation lies in the experiences that were matched between motor and sensory processes.

Understanding time and space relationships is important in understanding the concept of behavioral vision or behavioral low- vision care. When a mismatch of information occurs between sensory and motor processing, particularly vision and motor processing, distortions in experience occur. One theory is that these distortions are represented in the visual process as anomalies, i.e., myopia, hyperopia, astigmatism, malalignment of the eyes such as in strabismus, and particularly in the measurements of phorias (tendencies of variations of eye alignment that do not result in strabismus or eye turns). This is not to say that there are no other reasons for these anomalies. There can be organic and pathological causes. However, it is the author's clinical experience that all too often these anomalies, once diagnosed, are thought to be caused by an organic or pathological problem, and that the visual and functional cause related to motor and perceptual processing is often misdiagnosed. The purpose here is to emphasize the relationships of motor and sensory processes to the anomaly so that it may be analyzed in a new light and be dealt with by rehabilitative means.

Concerning any type of impairment, particularly a motor impairment, processing of information will be interfered with or distorted. Therefore, experience concerning time and space for a multihandicapped child will be affected because he will not be able to match information appropriately between the motor and sensory processes, particularly vision. Once again, we must question the appropriate mechanism of examination of a multihandicapped child, as well as the normally sighted child or the visually impaired child, with regard to sensory and motor testing. It is the author's opinion that the very states of esophoria and exophoria, myopia, astigmatism and hyperopia represent distortion and imbalances in time and space relationships as they occur in early stages of development. For example, if the child creates distortions in space because of inaccurate sensory-motor matching, then these distortions can also affect oculomotor balances that provide information to the brain about spatial relationships. This will be represented in the balance between the sensory component of the eyes and the ocular muscles, causing the eyes to overconverge to a closer point in space than where the person is actually fixating (esophoria). This means that the person will perceive the object in a different position than it really is. In the state of exophoria, individuals tend to see objects *farther* in space than they really are. Clinically, this behavior can be observed in patients diagnosed with a high state of esophoria or exophoria if they are given the opportunity to reach up and vertically point to an object in a touch-point situation. They will often reach up and touch a closer point than where the object actually is in the state of esophoria. In a state of high exophoria, when the person reaches up to touch the object, he will often touch beyond the object, indicating distortion in space.

Myopia and hyperopia may be looked at in a similar manner. Rather than distortions of ocular motor position, these conditions make distortions of focusing and sensory positions in space related to time concepts. For example, myopia is the tendency to focus at close points in space, blurring out distance. This pulls distance localization to near points in space.

Time and space relationships established through kinesthetic proprioceptive matching of information with the visual process become the basis for visual function. Any distortions that occur because of inaccurate matching may manifest as anomalies in the visual system. Over time, these distortions affect future judgments. The anomalies of visual development can be treated by changing perceptual and motor relationships affecting time and space judgments. When this occurs the anomaly of vision and very often the anomaly affecting motor dysfunction will be changed. This will be discussed in a more practical manner in the chapters devoted to assessment and treatment.

CHAPTER II

DEVELOPMENT OF THE VISUALLY IMPAIRED CHILD

The effects of both partial and total vision loss on the development of the child are examined in this chapter. Before delving into adaptations the child must make to a vision loss, a review of the development of the child with no visual impairment will be presented, as well as the importance of vision to normal development.

The discussion of developmental stages has been generally derived from research that includes observations of many children. The statements describing developmental stages are based upon norms in the population and are used to explain the developmental nature of the child. It must be understood that for every fact related to human maturation, there is an exception. With that in mind, the reader should use the text to form a broad understanding of development for the visually impaired child and the profound relationship of vision to development.

To understand the importance of the various senses in the perceptual development of the child, think of your own development. What is the very first experience that you can remember? Does it involve a visual experience, a motor experience, a tactual experience, an auditory experience, or a combination of sensory and motor experiences? How do you think the partially sighted or totally blind individual would respond to this question?

From this exercise you can begin to understand the function of individual senses in developing perceptual experiences. For most, I'm sure that the first thing that is remembered is a visual experience (seeing) with a secondary awareness of motor activity (doing). This illustrates the important relationship between the visual sense and early perceptual development.

The sighted newborn infant has a nondiscriminatory motor-sensory system. Observation of the newborn finds random motor activity that is uncoordinated and segmented. Just as arm and leg movements are uncoordinated, so are ocular movements. The child will glance momentarily at a moving object with monocular fixations. In a baby's development a rudimentary form of binocularity occurs at about eight weeks when he first fixates monocularly and then converges both eyes for momentary fixations. The infant now begins to develop a binocular space world through a reinforcement of vision and motor (eye-hand) coordination.

The maturing infant develops coordination of his motor and sensory functions through a process of utilizing sensory information to guide motor activity. The newborn infant has an undifferentiated motor and sensory system that begins to respond to sensory and motor information through reflexes and matching of information between sensory and motor processes at appropriate stages of development. The child must learn that his senses supply information that will yield economy and efficiency to his motor functioning. The process will involve learning how to control and manipulate the senses, while at the same time using motor reinforcement to make relationships.

The infant soon learns that his visual system will supply him with information about the environment that no other sense can. However, the visual process develops from the activities of a motor system. As Gesell so aptly stated, "Vision is an act mediated by eye and brain, although its development grows out of an action system."

The coordination of the visual-motor system permits the infant to begin to explore his environment. Visual-perceptual experiences develop from reinforcing vision with other motor-sensory experiences. The infant will prop himself on hands and knees and begin to creep at seven months. The creeping movements become a visual exploration of his environment. Eventually, the ability to stand erect at 10 months leads to walking at 12 months.

At this stage, motor activity is led by vision. The ability to maintain balance on two feet at 10 months is reinforced by matching information from the visual, vestibular and kinesthetic systems. These systems inform the child about position when he is perpendicular to the floor. Vision becomes more dominant as a sensory system as the child begins to walk. The visual system dynamically relays information about balance and movement, interrelating the motor and other sensory systems. However, as in crawling and creeping, the initial purpose of walking is to explore the environment, and this movement is stimulated and led by the visual sense.

The infant begins to trust his visual process as he develops visual perceptual experiences that are reinforced by the other senses: audition, touch and kinesthesia. Of the three million nerve impulses that travel to the brain each second, two-thirds are generated from the eye. Seventy percent of the sensory nerve fibers in the entire body originate from the eyes. From these statistics we can begin to understand the profound importance of the visual sense on the development of the child and the learning process.

The original question, "What is the first experience that you can remember?", can be related as a personal experience to this discussion. For most, there was a visual scene that may have involved an activity. It is important to note that the experience stemmed from a very early point in your development and, for most individuals, vision was the primary experience with some type of motor, auditory or tactual activity secondarily involved.

The Low-Vision Child

Suppose we were to ask a congenitally blind individual the same question about the very first experience that he can remember. How do you think his response would differ from the sighted or partially sighted individual? Since he would probably not be able to recount the experience visually, he would relate an auditory experience or a feeling. Also, if asked when this experience occurred, he may have more difficulty estimating the time period because there is no visualization of age or other experience to make a relative judgment. The experience that he recalls may be later in development compared to that of the sighted individual because the child formulates perceptual experiences from individual senses at different stages in his development. Since vision is the dominant process, a sighted child will most often use vision to develop his first experiences, relating the other senses to the visual experience. A congenitally blind child must learn to attend more formally to information received from the other senses. Since it is more difficult to initially utilize information from other senses to develop perceptual experiences such as object constancy, distance relationships, localization and direction, the child must wait for certain maturational levels before he can interpret the information and form perceptual relationships.

An interesting experiment by Friaberg, Siegel and Gibson showed that the normally sighted infant develops visual object constancy for a bell during the second quarter of his first year. In the experiment the low vision infant was unable to develop auditory object constancy until the last quarter of the first year. However, the low vision child was able to develop auditory object constancy to his mother's voice at the same age as the normally sighted child. Several factors may be involved. Under the experimental conditions, there was no survival instinct related to the bell. An infant does, however, learn to rely on his mother for nutrition and protection. If it is assumed that the newborn attends to auditory information for survival, he may develop auditory object constancy to tones important for survival but not for interest. A loud noise may indicate danger and initiate a crying response. The mother's voice signals warmth, nutrition, and protection and may initiate a smile. As a developmentally dominant sense, vision supplies information about survival and also allows the child to continually scan the environment for interest and stimulation. The sighted child may initially respond to a sound auditorily but will use his eyes to visually manipulate and reinforce information about the sound source. This ability to continually reinforce audition with vision and vice versa seems to help a normally sighted child develop the ability to maintain auditory object constancy at a younger age than the visually impaired child, who may have more difficulty reinforcing one sense with another.

From this discussion, it can be understood that perceptual experiences derived from the sensory-motor system are developmental in nature. Also, since vision is the dominant process, early perceptual experiences will develop mainly through reinforcement of the other senses and motor systems and vision. Because vision allows the child to manipulate and scan the environment, it will be the leading force to draw the child to the environment.

The blind child will prop himself on hands and knees at the same age (10 months) as the sighted child. However, the blind child will not advance himself by creeping until 12 months. Instead, the blind child will begin to rock back and forth, thereby replacing the visual stimulation with kinesthetic stimulation. Hence, the lack of vision interferes with the development of the infant. The delay in perceptual growth causes developmental lags. The chronological age of the child (age from birth) becomes a useless factor. The developmental age, or the age of the child based on his perceptual and physical abilities, should be emphasized. This concept not only applies to visually impaired children, but to all children.

Developmental lags are apparent and expected for the blind child. However, simply because a child has "normal" vision does not guarantee the absence of a developmental lag. The converse is also true; that is, a child suffering from an impairment, such as a vision loss, may not appear as developmentally delayed as another child with similar handicaps because he may be favored with a high intelligence quotient. He may use intellect to adapt himself and compensate for his handicap. Developmental lags are related to a variety of factors such as intelligence, environmental influences and physical abilities.

The visually impaired child, as all children, may skip a developmental stage and may even master an advanced stage early. Because of such factors as intelligence and physical abilities, the child may be able to formulate a relationship that is not expected until a later stage. Skipping a developmental stage does not infer that the child is advanced or that developmental age has no meaning. The child will show stages of rapid advancement, nonadvancement, and even remission that may be understood as cycles of development. However, a child that skips a developmental stage will eventually equalize himself in the cycles at some future point.

CHAPTER III

PERCEPTUAL DEVELOPMENT OF THE SIGHTED CHILD

To perceive, an individual must first be able to discern differences. If no differences are resolved, perceptual experience will be lacking or inappropriate.

The sighted infant can experience visual differences. He fixates on objects, pursues movement, and displays general visual attention. Different visual stimuli demand his attention. He may notice differences in brightness, color and movement. He may not, however, experience a perceptual difference in distances of two objects. Perceptual discrimination develops along with physical abilities, intelligence levels and environmental influences.

The infant's earliest visual attention is fixation on a light source. As the infant matures, he will fixate on objects and forms. Fixation represents a type of perception. He has discriminated a figure from the ground. He has recognized a contrast between two visual stimuli. The development of figure-ground perception is important because it marks the ability to discern visual relationships. With maturity and physical development, the infant utilizes figure-ground perception as a basis for developing other forms of perception.

As his motor coordination improves, the child will become intrigued by his extremities and his ability to control movement. Fixation on the hand is first noted during the *atonic necfk reflex (ATNR)* The head turns in the direction of the extended arm. When alternation of tonic neck reflex occurs, so does the fixation. The reinforcement of the kinesthetic awareness of arm extension with visual fixation gives the infant an awareness of his near-space world. As he gains greater control of his extremities and is able to manipulate objects, he begins to develop form perception and object constancy. Tactual manipulation of an object reinforces the visual manipulation of the same object. In turn, the child begins to transfer information from one sensory modality to another, ultimately building various perceptual experiences.

The child develops perceptual experience by extracting and analyzing information from the environment through his senses. The more able he is to extract information and discriminate similarities and differences of information received, the easier it will be for the child to build his perceptual experience. Many factors influence the development of the perceptual experience. Physical factors can interfere with the reception of information; emotional and psychological factors may interfere with both the ability to extract and analyze information. The analysis of information, of course, deals with meaning. Therefore, perception involves discerning relationships about information received in order to establish meaning.

Development of the Sighted Child
As the normally sighted infant develops, he shows increasing alertness and makes contact with the world through his vision. The infant learns to use his vision to guide his developing motor system. This is the most efficient and effective means for the infant to deal with his environment.

The functioning of the newborn's physiological and perceptual vision is peripheral, or ambient, in nature. The child will track an object as long as the movement of the object is beyond his central fixation. According to Trevarthen and Sperry (1973) there are two mechanisms of visual functioning: focal visual function and ambient visual function. For the infant the visual system functions primarily as a signal detection system. The evolution of such a process is, of course, for survival. Lower-order animals, which have not developed a focal ability, respond to movement as either a signal of impending danger or a food source.

Focal visual behavior matches information with the motor process with the development of the *atonic* neck reflex. At this point the infant is able to focus on the outstretched hand. This is the first time that he is able to match information received through one sensory modality (vision) with another (kinesthesia and proprioception). In the *ATNR* the child begins the process of restricting his visual awareness to a particular aspect of time and space rather than operating in the state of sensory scan. Over time, an ability to control the ambient and focal states will develop.

When the child has an ability to focalize and release with equal control, development will appear balanced and symmetrical. Increased focal ability will reciprocally develop during stages of asymmetry, i.e., a tonic neck reflex.

Table 1 summarizes the chronological visual development of the sighted child.

TABLE 1

DEVELOPMENT OF THE NORMALLY SIGHTED CHILD

Age	Visual Development
0-8 weeks	• Monocular visual fixations in ATNR • Spatially oriented ambient function • World segmented
8 weeks	• Begins to develop binocular control • Able to converge the eyes • Near-to-far fixations demonstrated • More focal in attention • Unable to fixate at midline
16 weeks	• Shows general awareness of environment • Stimulated by peripheral movement to direct central vision toward object • Fixations across midline show delay

20 weeks	• Itensified focal visual behavior with fixations on objects at near range • Fixations at midline improve • Eye-hand orientation control improves
24 weeks	• Able to team eye-hand responses • When seizing object with hand, child will bring it to mouth (refining form and substance perception).
28 weeks	• Immediately releases object after touching lips (evidence of developing perceptual constancy) • Demonstrates general awareness of surroundings
32 weeks	• Able to localize auditory sounds by directing visual fixation on sound source • Focalization extends to more distant environment • Seems unable to deal with tri-dimensionality of space; instead, segments space and seems to look at an object moved from one position to another as a completely new object.
40 weeks	• Deals with the world as a whole • Rises to hands and knees and begins to creep • Visual attention diminishes as child explores new balance and visual-motor relationships
12 months	• Rises to feet and begins to walk • Focalization that began to appear for short period disappears as child explores visual-motor relationships • After balance improves, the child will again develop interest in detail and will focalize visual function • Looks back and forth between hand and object when attempting to grasp object

15 months	• Becomes more aware of relationship between sight and sound • Visually focuses on the object he intends to grasp rather than between hand and object
18 months	• Driven by motor movement • Ambient visual function • Attention fleeting • Able to build blocks vertically
21 months	• Visual focal behavior • Actively looking and visually intense • Visually cautious • Balance falters • Gives thought to visual situations and appears to ponder situation before becoming involved
2 years	• Predilection for small objects • Focal behavior continues • Develops dimension of language to visual-spatial dimensions • Increased eye-hand coordination
2 1/2 years	• Easily distractible • Very peripheral • Increased ability to discern relationships between other senses and vision (using past experiences)
3 years	• Plans in advance • More attentive to eye-hand coordination • Central in attention • Able to confine to boundaries and draw rather than scribble
3 1/2 years	• Becomes uncertain and anxious about abilities • Clings for protection • Fear of high places

4 years	• Understands symmetry • Very assertive • Sees part-to-whole relationship • Seems to shift from one thing to another
5 years	• Greater stability and much more in charge of situation • Deals with one thing at a time • Greater ability to make vertical strokes than horizontal • Able to match according to size and shape
6 years	• Appears clumsy • Becomes unsure of himself • Attempts oblique stroke • Eruptive behavior
7 years	• Withdrawn and pensive • Lacks self-limits • Easily frustrated • Prints smaller
8 years	• Expansive • Increased social behavior • Grasps totality

In the first eight weeks the visual system of the sighted infant has not developed coordination of binocular fixations. Just as his motor movements are erratic and show lack of control, so are his eye movements. Fixation is monocular, and unilateral divergence and convergence movements are seldom observed. Because the infant is still exhibiting the atonic neck reflex, monocular eye fixation to his outstretched hand may occur. As the infant shifts from the left to the right side, fixation often changes from one eye to the other. His visual world is segmented.

At eight weeks of age the sighted infant begins to develop enough control to binocularly align his eyes to fixate and converge. This establishes new spatial relationships since there is a transition from near to far through the convergence and divergence of the eyes. The infant at this age is intrigued by bright objects like flaming candles and increases his attention to the object when it is moved.

By 16 weeks the infant begins to respond to his visual world as if he were experiencing a new setting. He shifts his attention, showing an increased awareness. Fixation changes are easier for the infant when he is in the supine position.

At 20 weeks fixation intensifies and the infant focuses on objects placed within a near range at chest-high level. He watches objects at his midline with increasing efficiency. Before this period, visual fixations across the midline showed delays of eye movements or loss of fixations. The coordination of binocular fixations on the midline permit the child to improve head manipulations, and by 24 weeks he is able to team eye-hand responses.

When the infant seizes an object with his hands, it is drawn immediately to his mouth. This response indicates that he is developing perception of form and substance. The infant is reinforcing visual information with tactual information. As his visual perceptual experiences are reinforced by other senses, he will no longer need this added input to derive meaningful information about an object. By 24 weeks the infant immediately releases the object upon touching it to his lips. He relies on his visual interpretation of the object and has less need for other sensory reinforcement. The infant is more inspectional.

By the age of 32 weeks the infant is able to localize sounds beyond his reach. This ability reinforces the infant's visual projections into his space environment. He is still unable to conceive the tri-dimensionality of his environment. He needs additional experiences to develop depth perception. However, the 36-week-old infant shows better orientation in space.

At 40 weeks the infant responds to the totality of a situation. He views the world as a whole rather than an isolated or segmented portion. Development continues in a series of cycles. When a cycle is repeated, the infant uses his newly acquired abilities to examine his environment in a new way. New perceptual experiences are developed. In contrast to the 32-week-old infant, the cycles of development have brought the 40-week-old to a more focalized regard of his environment. At this age the infant can be observed to shift objects obliquely. This is a method of exploiting and reorganizing his perceptions of space. Spatial exploration through motor movement and visual pervasion progressively constructs a perceptual model or an interpretation of the three-dimensional domain. At the age of 40 weeks the infant begins to explore the relationships of three dimensions.

By one year the child shows a basic understanding of his three-dimensional domain. At this age he shows auditory perception of distant objects. It appears that the basic understanding of three-dimensional space develops through an interweaving of multisensory experiences. The child is able to sight an object visually, reinforce the sighting with motor movement involving tactile and kinesthetic input, and also integrate auditory perception of sounds with visual and motor perception of distance. Spatial perception is also observed with the child's ability to move objects alongside or above another object.

The one-year-old child shows increased interest in small objects such as buttons and buckles. At this age he appears intrigued with the permeability of his space world and shows interest in placing objects through holes. There is also an awareness of emotions perceived through facial expressions. The child may begin to imitate these expressions.

At 15 months the child becomes more acutely aware of the relationships between sights and sounds. He demonstrates interest in following moving objects or people, particularly if there are accompanying sounds. The child's motor movement and hand manipulations have continued to improve. At one year of age, when the child wanted to place an object in something else, he picked up the object and watched his hand move toward the final position. As the hand approached the final position, correctional movements would then be made to bring the object into the desired position. The 15-month-old child grasps the object but looks at the point toward which he is directing his movement.

The child's development proceeds with a purpose to maximize efficiency within his environment. Vision as the dominant sense allows the child maximum efficiency and a conservation of energy. Because of this, the child allows vision to lead motor movement.

By 18 months the child is strongly driven by motor movement. This drive is so strong that it appears as if the motor is leading vision. The child is occupied by the present, and his attention appears to flit from one activity or thing to another. At this age he is able to build blocks vertically but has difficulty arranging them horizontally.

Growth is rapid during the next several months, and by 21 months the child's behavior and perceptions of the world have changed dramatically. Vision is dominant and the child is both visually alert and visually tense. He approaches activities and people with caution. His spatial orientation to the environment, particularly in new areas, becomes much more tentative. There appears to be more thought given to situations where only a few months earlier he seemed to act with little thought given to the consequences.

By two years the child may have a fascination for small objects. At this age he uses words such as "where" to gain information concerning spatial perception. The ability to decode language by hearing it spoken allows the child to reinforce perceptual experiences. Like all of the child's perceptual experiences, meaningful language is concrete and does not deal with abstraction of an object or a situation. At two years there is also increased eye-hand coordination. Although fine motor tremors are still observed, the child has adequate control over gross movements.

The two-and-one-half-year-old child is easily distracted. The slightest movement in his peripheral vision will capture his attention. The best method to hold this child's attention on a task is to keep him involved manually and visually. At this age he has difficulty planning ahead; he is still occupied by the here and now. The two-and-one-half-year-old demonstrates increasing ability to discern differences through vision and other senses. This is an important development because the child uses past experiences to examine relationships. If the relationships about an object or situation are not detectable as a difference, then the child will interpret them as the same, such as when a child cannot feel the difference between a rectangular shape and a square shape, or when he has reversals in writing.

At the age of three, unlike the two-and-one-half-year-old, the child will plan in advance and show greater organizing ability. Eye-hand coordination is more accurate, and the child is not so distracted. He is more central in his attention, as observed in his paper and pencil work. He can confine himself to boundaries while drawing, whereas six months earlier he scribbled all over the paper. The three-year-old also shows a preoccupation with the wholeness of things, or perceptual closure. He tries to organize things in symmetrical relationships and will become upset when the organization is broken.

By three-and-one-half years the child becomes uncertain of his abilities, anxious of new situations, and tends to cling for protection. He appears to view things in a segmented manner, and the organized holistic qualities previously exhibited seem lost in the child's confusion about relationships and parts. He will indicate a fear of high places and will appear generally clumsy.

By four years old the child again perceives symmetry in relationships. He has become very assertive, and the introspective qualities of the three-and-one-half-year-old have disappeared. His perception of the whole continues, but he is now also able to see the parts of a whole and the whole as parts.

The five-year-old seems more stable than the four-year-old. He appears much more in charge of things and knows his limits. He prefers dealing with one thing at a time and enjoys the accomplishment of finishing a task. The child knows enough control to make vertical and horizontal strokes but is still unable to draw an oblique line. These perceptual patterns are related to the maturation level of his oculomotor system. The five-year-old also discriminates according to size, position and form. He can demonstrate perceptual constancy by matching or grouping by size and form, but prefers to position in a vertical line. He is able to see parts without separating them from the whole.

Within a few months' time the static and stable five-year-old turns into a reactive, unstable six-year-old. This eruptive period marks a transition to a more complete and controlled child. The child often suffers from physical ailments, allergies and frequent infections. His motor behavior may be very clumsy, and binocular coordination shows fluctuations and momentary monocular shifts. The child will attempt to master the oblique stroke and demonstrate a variety of body shifts and paper rotations.

By seven the child's eruptive behavior dissipates, and he becomes a more stable personality. The seven-year-old is withdrawn and pensive. Thought precludes actions, and he appears to be reorganizing his thought processes and experiences. The visual process actively engages thought, experiences and interpretation of information while it guides motor responses. Through self-organization the child develops habits that may appear somewhat fanatical. He carries himself to the extremes of a task and lacks self-limits. The frustrations observed are an indication of inner tension and conflict. With this characteristic self-control, the child will also begin to print smaller.

The eight-year-old is expansive, similar to the six-year-old. The child moves out on all levels. He is increasingly social and demonstrates strong need for peer companionship. The eight-year-old draws from the organizational skills he developed as a seven-year-old as he learns to commit himself by drawing conclusions. He is able to grasp the totality of situations and work through tasks without making imposing short-term goals or limits necessary.

There are increased gross and fine motor coordination skills exhibited. His writing becomes more balanced and uniform, and his drawing indicates an increasing awareness of perspective relationships. This appears to be related to improved time and space orientation. In grasping the totality of space and the relationship to time, the child shows increasing ease in shifting from near to far activities. This differs from the seven-year- old, who could work in only one plane, near or far, at a time. At this level the child also develops the concept of directionality.

The nine-year-old shows a growing sense of self-awareness, motivation and responsibility. He seeks responsibility and follows through on tasks. Expansiveness is counterbalanced by self-awareness as he realizes that the frontiers to explore are not only in the external world. He focuses attention on one activity at a time, an important implication for the educator.

By the age of 10 he becomes less focused in attention and is more able to deal with his new self-awareness and the external world simultaneously. The 10-year-old, like the 5-year-old, is realistic, seeks accomplishment, and is well-oriented in his world. In general, he is a more balanced individual.

CHAPTER IV

PERCEPTUAL DEVELOPMENT OF THE VISUALLY IMPAIRED CHILD

Considering that the normally sighted child may manifest a developmental lag, it should be apparent that a partial impairment to sight alone does not cause a developmental lag. The partially sighted child may utilize a variety of sensory-motor abilities to compensate for and eventually adapt to his visual impairment. There is no direct relationship between partial sight loss (impairment) and a lag in development.

Sight refers to the eye and optic nerve sending information to the cortex. Vision refers to the dynamic process of matching information between sight and other sensory-motor modalities. The matching process is not passive. It is an active manipulation and examination of the details of our environment. The relationship of these details understood through this matching process forms a perception of the environment that is unique to each individual. When a child is unable to compensate for and adapt to sight loss, the matching process is affected. A developmental lag occurs because vision has been interfered with. The relationship between sight and development is an indirect one, but vision is directly related to development.

The low vision infant who is sight-impaired does not manifest predictable delays in development. He may demonstrate all the expected developmental milestones. Even more profoundly, for sight-impaired children who have manifested developmental lags, the percentage of sight loss does not equal the percentage of vision loss.

Figure 1 displays a model of child development. The three legs of the pyramid represent the main supports of child development: physical attributes, psychological disposition (intelligence, personality, etc.), and environmental surroundings. The arrows at the base of the pyramid indicate the interaction of the three variables with each other. If one of the legs is affected (see Figure 2), it depends upon the other two areas to compensate for the deficit.

Sight is physical. Vision encompasses physical attributes and psychological disposition and is stimulated by the environment. A child with a sight impairment who has above average intelligence and a stimulating environment may be able to maintain a keen enough state of visual awareness and function to compensate for and adapt to the sight loss and not manifest any delay in development. On the other hand, a developmental delay may occur in an older child if the demands are greater than the child's ability to compensate and adapt. In the latter case, vision is affected, thereby causing a developmental lag. The likelihood of manifesting a developmental lag at the various developmental stages will, of course, vary from child to child.

A developmental lag may be determined through observation of behavior. However, to accurately test, diagnose and classify the problem would require an experienced analyst. Since it is not the scope of this text to give detailed methods of testing and scoring, it is suggested that the

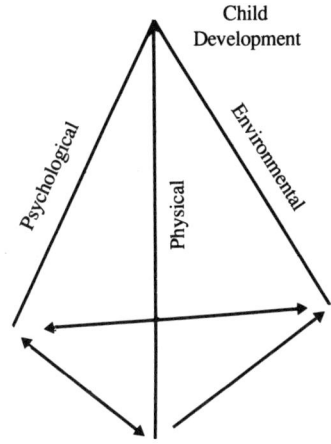

Figure 1. Child development demonstrated as a relationship between physical, psychological and environmental variables.

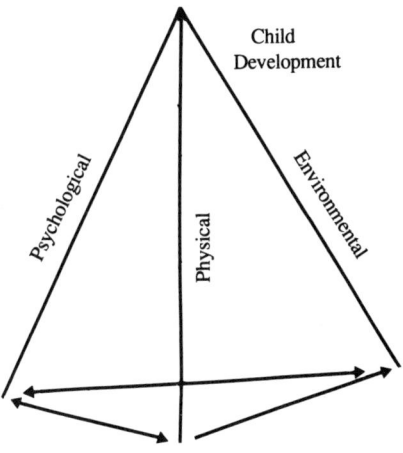

Figure 2. Abnormal child development demonstrated by variations in support between physical, psychological and environmental variables.

reader refer to the sources listed in the bibliography for specific tests, methods of testing, and means of analysis.*

*An excellent diagnostic assessment procedure is the "Program to Develop Efficiency in Visual Functioning," developed by Natalie Barraga, Ed.D., and Marcia Collins, Ed.D. Visual tasks as they relate to normal developmental milestones are outlined. In addition, the developmental milestones are broken down into optical, perceptual and visual perceptual functions to enable the instructor to obtain more specific assessment data. The complete assessment/diagnostic series is available through the American Printing House for the Blind. It is an invaluable assessment tool for the teacher involved in evaluation of children with low vision.

This information would apply to the visually handicapped adult. The optical difficulties inherent in using aids will decrease perceptual interpretations of visual stimuli. More studies are needed with the adult to determine what specific parameters of development and perception are "altered," but it must be obvious that there is an important relationship.

Development of the Blind Child

The development of the blind or visually impaired child will proceed in a manner similar to the sighted child, but the lack of visual influence will show developmental lags. Just as normally sighted children have varying developmental lags because of different genetic, environmental and psychological backgrounds, blind and partially sighted children will also exhibit developmental lags. The amount of developmental lag is not directly proportional to the amount of acuity or field loss.

Table 2 summarizes the development of the totally blind child between birth and five years of age.

The discussion of development for the blind child is limited to the age of five because the variations in the child's ability to adapt and compensate for the lack of vision increases with age. Therefore, the accuracy of any developmental schedule for the visually impaired child becomes more difficult to predict.

TABLE 2

DEVELOPMENT OF THE BLIND CHILD

Age	Visual Development
16 weeks	• Hands to midline • Facial expressions • Searching eye movements • Auditorily attentive to familiar sounds • Exaggerated limb movement
28 weeks	• Transfers objects from one hand to the other • Hand preference may be noted • Shows greater recognition to familiar sounds • Greater oral tendencies for blind child • Tendency for prolonged rubbing of eyes • Sitting up may be delayed due to lack of visual interest and support; this will develop in several weeks.
40 weeks	• Uses tactual and auditory cues to explore objects • Demonstrates interest with feet • Expresses first words • Props on hands and knees but does not creep; rocks back and forth
12 months	• Accurate scissors grasp • Strong motor drive by creeping • Continues to show curiosity with feet • Rocks continuously in seated position • Localizes sounds by directing hand toward sound source • Stands only if prompted

15 months	• Walks with one hand held • Gait is wide-spread with short steps
18 months	• Walks for brief periods • Easily disoriented • Will drop to floor to regain orientation • Unable to use sound for orientation • Releases objects into cup and retrieves them • Lacks understanding of three-dimensional space • Begins to develop concept of distance through audition and tactual-motor reinforcement • Developing object constancy
24 months	• Walks with greater control • Walks toward familiar sounds and voices • Able to use sounds for orientation • Tactually inquisitive
30 months	• Able to identify shapes of familiar objects • Uses sound to explore consistency of objects and to further develop concepts of time and distance
3 years	• Begins to match information between motor movement and audition to develop three-dimensional concept of space • Improved motor-coordination and balance seems to keep the child motorically bound and very much aware of peripheral sounds • Able to construct vertical row of blocks with one hand
4 years	• Appears to regress in many areas • Timing and coordination falter • Anxious and cautious of new situations • Seems unable to cope with more than one action at a time • Peripheral sounds or activities can cause frustration with the activity at hand

	• Segmented understanding of space • Appears disorganized
5 years	• Has developed a concept of body symmetry and, when touching body parts of another person, will search for corresponding eye or arm, etc. • Motor-coordination improves • Seems more in control of situations and likes to be actively involved.

The 16-week-old blind infant will meet most of the diagnostic developmental norms of the sighted infant (see Table 1). However, deviations in behavior will be noted as a result of his visual loss. The blind child will bring his hands to his midline and demonstrate active, spontaneous fingering of his hands. This is also seen in sighted infants. When the child expresses excitement he will breath heavily and laugh spontaneously. The blind child will also demonstrate a searching or groping type of pursuit movement with his eyes when attempting to locate objects with his hands. The blind infant may appear to listen more than the sighted child.

Although all developmental norms in the blind child are met at this stage, various motor movements and postures may be observed that are different from those of the sighted child. Head rotations may appear restricted, and there may be exaggerated movements of the head and limbs. Both sighted and non-sighted children will cease all movement upon hearing a familiar sound or voice. It appears as if the child is attempting momentarily to suppress all other sensory stimuli, including vision for the sighted child, to direct his attention to sound. The primary difference will be that the sighted child will then attempt to direct his vision to the sound, thereby allowing him to transfer information between sensory modalities.

At 28 weeks the blind child continues to meet developmental norms. He will transfer objects from one hand to the other and on a tactile cue will reach out for an object with one hand. A hand preference may be noted at this time. His hands will be open more than during previous ages. He is able to roll to a prone position. At this age the child will also begin to show greater recognition and partiality to certain sounds that have become important to him.

The child will lift his head from the supine position and should be able to sit erect momentarily and support his weight when in a standing position. However, due to the lack of visual stimulation, motor development such as sitting and standing may not appear at this time. Since the child lacks vision, he may not be interested in sitting or standing. Within a short time this behavior should change.

At this age the blind infant will show greater oral tendencies than the sighted child. He may often touch his tongue with his fingers. Mouthing of objects allows the blind child to reinforce tactile experiences concerning form and substance. As his sense of touch becomes more developed, he will have less need to gain information by mouthing objects. Other deviant behaviors may include frequent and prolonged rubbing of his eyes.

By 40 weeks the blind child will, on tactual and auditory cues, explore a small object with his index finger and pick it up with a pincer grasp. He will also show an interest in his feet and will play with them often. His expansion at this age into the near environment also leads him to exploration of distant parts of his body. His first words (mama, dada) are usually spoken at this age, and he becomes more social. He will be aware of disapproval and will become upset when scolded.

The sighted child at this age will creep on hands and knees about his crib or the floor. The blind child will prop himself up on his hands and knees but will not begin to creep. Instead, he will rock back and forth. Since he lacks visual stimulation, he has no need to move forward, so he will seek kinesthetic stimulation by rocking. Any forward creeping movements will be a consequence of seeking kinesthetic stimulation. The age of 10 months usually marks the first sign of a lag in development, and it clearly relates to visual loss. The child will sit up straight but will not pull himself to a standing position unless helped. His postures and movements, particularly in the prone position, although better coordinated than at 28 weeks, will still appear disjointed and impulsive. He will continue to mouth his hands and objects with more than normal frequency.

The one-year-old blind infant will show an accurate scissors grasp and transfer from one hand to the other. He will not be satisfied by only listening but will demonstrate a stronger motor drive. He will creep without prompting and, in general, will show an exploring behavior. With prompting and support, the child will stand and take a step or two. In the supine position he will continue to show curiosity for his feet. In the seated position he will rock constantly. He will localize sounds and direct hand movement. This marks an important phase in the child's development of spatial perception.

By 15 months he will walk with one hand held and begin to walk by himself. His gait will be widespread, and his steps will be short. To maintain maximum balance the child may shuffle along the floor.

The 18-month-old child will walk about the room for brief periods. If he does not come into contact with any objects, he will seek orientation by dropping to the floor. The three-dimensional space world through which he walks is boundless. The child should be encouraged to walk and investigate. Tactual stimulation, such as placing a large ball at the child's feet, will give him a sense of direction and orientation. As he shuffles his feet forward, he will come into constant contact with the ball as he dribbles it across the floor.

The child will also be able to drop objects into a cup and retrieve them. He will remain alert to auditory and tactile clues about his spatial environment. He will approach stairs and investigate them with caution. His comprehension of the steps in three-dimensional space is lacking; therefore, he will not attempt to climb them. The child will be able tactually to discriminate various geometric forms. A form box could be used to encourage the child to explore and retrieve different shapes from within the box. When the form is placed in the correct hole and falls in, the child experiences a tactile loss and hears the sound of the object as it falls into the box.

The association of the tactual loss and sound will develop object constancy in the child.

Since he does not have visual abilities to manipulate and investigate his environment and develop various forms of perception, the child will, through sensory transfer, reinforce sensory information to construct his perceptual models. At this age the child will overturn a cup to find a hidden cube that was previously presented to the child both tactually and auditorily. This is further evidence of the development of object constancy.

By the age of 24 months the child is able to stand and walk with greater facility, although his posture is rigid, stance wide and steps small. Sounds and familiar voices will stimulate the child to walk in that general direction. The child will take several steps and stop, attempting to reorganize information for orientation and direction. He may also squat intermittently to bring himself in contact with the floor to gain stability.

The child will begin to explore and may climb several stairs. This may be very disorienting to him since he has previously explored only flat planes such as the floor. The blind child lives in a flat, two-dimensional world. His visual deficit does not allow him to view the world from different perspectives; his only contact is through tactual and auditory means. When the child is picked up, he loses contact with his reference plane. He has no idea of the distance which he has traveled to his parent's shoulder because he has no relative reference plane.

By 24 months the child will build several wide blocks vertically. For that activity he should be encouraged to use one hand to gain information about the position and location of the tower of blocks. Blocks may be introduced by tapping them on the table to give him a sound cue. At this age he will be more tactually inquisitive and will show random motor movement.

The 30-month-old blind child will identify the shapes of familiar objects such as a ball or box by manipulating them. After he has identified the object, he will shake it briefly with one hand and then release it. The sound of the object hitting another surface is then associated with the release of the object from the hand. In that way, the child begins to build a time and space relationship without active movement from one place to another. Previously in his development, time and space relationships were formulated by an active motor movement such as creeping or walking from one position to another. By approximately 30 months the child will begin to explore the environment, using himself as a reference point. His horizon will be extended from the limits of his reach to the limits of sounds which he can create by throwing an object.

By three years of age the child will begin to examine his relationship with the ground below him. He will take objects placed on a table in front of him and move them to the edge of the table where he will release them. From the sound of the objects coming into contact with the floor, the child further constructs his perception of the three-dimensional world. When the object is retrieved for the child, he will respond by duplicating the act, much to the dismay of his kind-hearted teacher. It may appear as if the child is purposely attempting to be aggravating; however, the simple retrieval of the object has fascinated him. From the retrieval, he has learned the permanence of things. There are limits to his world, and sounds created by objects coming into contact with another surface represent a limit on structure to his environment.

At three years the child will sit erect but will show exaggerated head movements. When manipulating an object, he will rotate his head into various positions while rolling his eyes in a random movement. His coordination has improved to the extent that he can pedal a tricycle and delight in the sensation.

The four-year-old in many respects will appear to regress in development. His timing and coordination will fault. He may also become very cautious and show fear in activities that he accomplished with no difficulty six months previously. He will become frustrated and even rebellious at certain tasks.

The four-year-old's conceptualization of space is segmented. At an earlier age (three years old), he was able to construct a tower of blocks at his midline using one hand to locate the position and the other to place them. At four years old the child will attempt to build them with both hands. He loses the relationship of one block to another. His concept of the whole has been temporarily disorganized. This is a period of regrouping and reorganizing perceptual experiences and skills.

The rapid advancements in perceptual development during the first four years of the blind child's life closely parallel that of the normal child. Because of his visual deficit, developmental lags occur. Those lags will vary from month to month. The child may appear to be developmentally behind six months at one age and then show almost no lag when observed at another age. At one age the child may be unable to utilize other sensory information in place of his vision to create a particular perceptual experience, and a lag occurs in development. Within a few months the child is able to utilize the same information in a new way that becomes meaningful to him, such as utilizing another sense in place of his vision. This allows him to establish the perceptual experience. Upon establishing this experience and finding a new way to examine his environment, he may decrease his developmental lag in a relatively short period of time. From five to nine years of age the development of the blind child will be more stable in advancement but will show fluctuations according to his particular developmental level. The developmental lag should also stabilize. It becomes apparent that the first four years are perhaps the most important of the blind child's life. It is during this time that he constructs the framework which he can build on later.

CHAPTER V

DEFINING THE IMPAIRMENT AND DEVELOPING A MODEL OF SERVICES

By understanding the major influence of vision on development, we can be more effective in designing therapeutic programs for children and rehabilitation programs for impaired individuals. It is important to examine the use of current terminology as it relates to any impairment to increase uniformity within the field for classification and treatment.

The most commonly used terminology describing vision afflictions include: visually impaired, visually handicapped, low vision individuals, sight deprived, partially sighted, legally blind, blind and sight impaired. These are often very misleading, and vary in popularity according to geography and from one agency to another. The federal government sometimes sets trends through the use of various descriptive terms in existing legislation and grants.

Because of misconceptions concerning what vision is, finding a single general term to describe the anomaly of impairment has not been a simple task. The most popular terms presently used are visually handicapped and visually impaired. However, the use of the word "visually" implies a condition well beyond the scope of present standardized testing, diagnosis and treatment.

The standards set by the Department of Health and Human Services for determining the proper classification of visually impaired, legally blind and blind stem from the measurements of the individual's visual acuity and visual field. The definition of legally blind states that a person must have a visual acuity of "20/200 in the best-corrected eye or less than a 20 degree visual field." Typically, "20/70 or less in the best-corrected eye" is the standard for partially sighted, visually handicapped or visually impaired.

These definitions describe measurements that are taken during an eye examination and may not describe how the individual functions in his environment. The visual acuity and the visual field measurements indicate the impairment to the eyeball and to the individual's sight but do not necessarily indicate functional- perceptual abilities.

The static measurements of visual acuity and visual fields are measurements of eyesight. Vision, on the other hand, is a process by which visual input is related to motor movement, balance, thought process, endocrine function, metabolism or any other action within the body. The relationship is not a one-way process but an interchange between motor, sense, thought and physiology which influences function and perception. Vision, therefore, is a dynamic process and should be analyzed as such.

An individual with an impairment to his acuity or field has an impairment to his sight but may not be impaired visually. The converse is also true; an individual may not be sight-impaired but may have interferences causing deficits in visual abilities. The impairment to sight may cause impairment to vision; however, visual impairment is not to be expected by the measurements of acuity or field, but only anticipated. The extent of visual impairment cannot be measured by only acuity or field.

Technically, it is appropriate to classify a person who has lowered acuity or a reduced field as sight impaired. Unfortunately, any classification of impairment tends to label the negative aspects of a person's condition as opposed to the positive aspects. Describing the individual as exceptionally sighted might eliminate negative connotation and thereby allow an accent on his capabilities. However, under present modes of classification, "sight impairment" is the correct terminology describing affliction to acuity and/or field.

The term low vision is presently used very broadly. It describes the concept or general classification under which other classifications and services are provided and should not be used to classify the individual. Measurements taken in testing to determine the low vision classification really determine only sight impairment.

The type of treatment most commonly available to those with sight impairment is the low vision examination. This includes testing of sight and the prescription of optical aids to improve sight. These aids are very important to the rehabilitation of the sight- impaired individual, but there are many individuals who receive various optical aids and are not successful in using them. Providing that the aids have been accurately prescribed, the reason for the lack of success is the inability of the individual to adapt his visual processes to accommodate the optical aid. For these visually impaired individuals a new area of the low vision field needs to be developed and explored. The author calls this area "low vision utilization" or "low vision efficiency." It involves developing the use of the process of vision, not just eyesight.

Within the area of low vision utilization, some professionals have already begun investigation and treatment. Terms such as vision stimulation, visual efficiency and visual functioning have been used to describe the programs that have been developed to improve the visual abilities of visually impaired individuals. Training in how to use the optical aid is also included in this category.

Because of the importance vision has to the development and learning process, most of the work that has been developed in this area has been directed toward children. Much more investigation into new techniques and methods of treatment is needed. Programs to improve visual abilities in adults has, in general, been overlooked by the low vision field.

The concept of low vision as presented here is divided into several phases. The examination, which should be performed by a qualified eye-care professional, such as an optometrist and/or an ophthalmologist, involves analyzing the health status, sight loss and optical aids needed to improve sight. Since these eye-care professionals most often will not see the individual in his habitual environment, information concerning how the person functions and uses his vision (low vision utilization) should be collected by professionals who can analyze the individual's behaviors in the field. Social workers, orientation and mobility specialists, rehabilitation specialists, occupational and physical therapists, audiologists, teachers and other professionals should determine the functional-perceptual visual difficulties. These specialists should observe behavior, not measure visual acuities or visual fields.

The information gathered by professionals in an individual's habitual environment could include answers to questions such as: Does the individual attempt to use his vision? How does the individual turn his head in a particular way when using his vision? What are the perceptive abilities? How does the person learn?

For example, the following information was provided regarding Patient A, a 40-year-old male businessman, a 20/800 best-corrected distance acuity with 10 degree binocular field: (Patient A) was able to see a black felt-tip pen on a desk top at 35 cm but had difficulty locating it with his right hand. In order to write, he had to hold his head within 5 cm of the paper. The 75-watt bulb in the goose-neck lamp he had placed directly in front of himself appeared to have a relationship to the increased blinking, squinting and watering eyes that occurred when he attempted to write. When Patient A attempted to scan the environment to visually locate an audible sound, he consistently overshot the target. Head movements were used with little or no eye movements observed during saccadic fixations (a quick change of visual fixation). When reaching for an object, Patient A turned his head to the right while still fixating, but showed little ability to utilize visual information regarding depth and localization. The behavior noted was a tactile searching with his right hand.

This information enabled the examiner to take a direct approach to the low vision examination and also alerted him to the visual and perceptual difficulties and needs of the individual. A possible glare problem and/or extreme light sensitivity observed during near working conditions was noted. The examiner was made aware that Patient A had spatial perception difficulty, and that he was unable to establish the necessary spatial relationships by matching information received through various sensory modalities. Distance-magnification devices, which further limit the field of view, would most likely cause more disorientation in this individual. The examination was oriented to improving near vision through optical aids. Therapy was recommended to improve spatial perceptions and scanning techniques with the intention of readying Patient A for distance magnification devices.

Behavioral assessments should be developed by professionals who are involved in the rehabilitation of the individual along with ongoing active communication with the examiner. All too often when a patient is referred, the examiner is unaware of the specific needs of the individual, and inappropriate optical aids are sometimes prescribed. The converse also occurs when aids are prescribed without the professionals in the field knowing why. Ideally, there would be a team approach to documenting information concerning a patient's needs based on abilities of sight and low vision utilization. Any recommended aids and/or therapy could be designed by an interdisciplinary approach and initiated by the instructors.

The model of services described here is not the only way to achieve the philosophy, definitions and general approach outlined in this paper. This chapter is meant to alert the reader to the present state of low vision services and to stimulate thought regarding further improvement of these services. This could increase the efficiency and success ratio for the sight- and visually impaired person. The challenge to apply this concept lies not with one profession, but with all professions associated with the field of low vision.

CHAPTER VI

POSTURAL DEVELOPMENT AND VISION

At birth an infant enters a gravity-based environment. In order to cope with this new existence the baby must develop an ability to right his body in space. Righting responses occur at an automatic level of the central nervous system and start with the lifting of the head off the surface. This is more than a life-saving reaction to keep the air passages of the infant cleared when he is in the prone position. Its importance to our understanding of the interrelationship between postural control and vision is that the weight of the head on the nose and mouth causes a reaction in the extensor musculature of the neck, which in turn causes the infant to lift his head off the surface.

The early and automatic turning of the face to one side already offers the newborn infant a change of visual environment. That postural response is also creating an opportunity for the visual system to begin to organize the three-dimensional world parallel to the postural reactions to gravity. Although there is some light perception in utero, we might think of the discriminative features of vision beginning at birth as well.

During the first few weeks of life the normal infant makes a systematic effort to develop extension of the body that moves him away from the physiological flexion with which he was born. In the prone, or face down, position he stretches his legs out one at a time as his pelvis shifts from one side to another. His center of gravity is forward at this stage of development, with the body weight sustained over the sternum and chest. Early arm support is characterized by the elbows being at the level of the chest. The long extensor muscles of the back lift the head and shoulders as a unit away from the surface, which in turn permits the arms to move forward gradually in a more versatile support of the torso. Each of these changes brings the face a little closer to a perpendicular alignment in relation to the base of support, what Gesell identified as a "level three" head lift. Visual interest contributes significantly to the maintenance of uprightness, which is sustained a little longer each time.

It is characteristic of normal development that movement occurs away from the surface, that is, against gravity, which is perceived by the organism as a pleasant challenge and acts as a stimulus for normal reflexive movements. The child with neuromotor dysfunction can be identified as the infant who fails to accept the challenge of gravity and is seen to be caught in its pull instead of moving away from its influence. The dysfunctioning baby will have difficulty lifting the head and shifting over the longitudinal midline of the body.

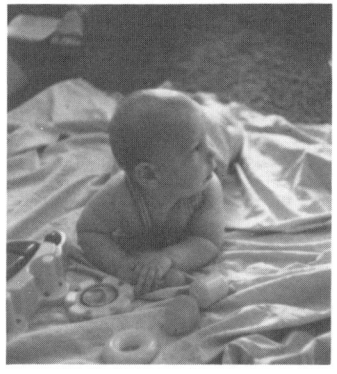

A. *Vision and posture. Normal postural control supports visual exploration.*

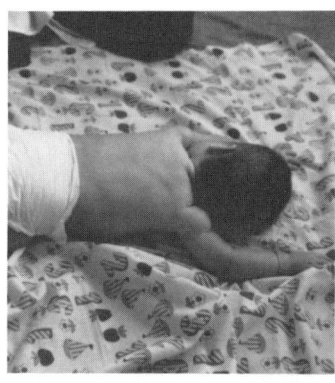

B. *Prone without extension. Lack of back extension and inactive legs are causes for concern in baby development.*

A lateral shift of weight is essential to organize the musculature of the trunk for postural control. The baby prepares himself with many subtle weight changes to support his body over one side while he reaches for a toy with the opposite hand. Initially, he overbalances just as he visually misjudges the distance to an object. By seven months, however, the active baby is able to pivot in the prone position to obtain a toy placed at his side, an accomplishment that represents a significant level of integration of vision and posture. It is an important step in the establishment of bilaterality, which is essential for the sensory organization of vision, audition and learning by the central nervous system.

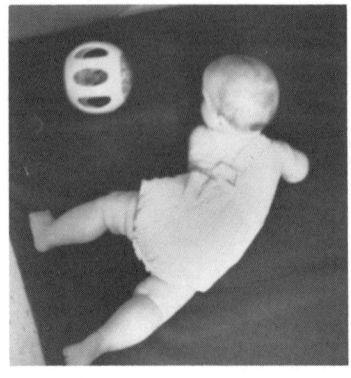

C. Pivot prone. Lateral flexion of the trunk in the "pivot prone" response corresponds with lateral eye movement.

Early changes in postural orientation from one side of the body to the other begin to integrate the longitudinal midline as one arm is used to reach and the other to support body weight. This early turning of the body is accomplished by a lengthening of the side that maintains the body weight and a shortening of the moving side. It reflects the interaction of stability and mobility so essential for smooth movement reactions. Although this maneuver is already seen in the baby of six or seven months of age, it is a sign of developmental preparation for the distant ability of taking a step forward with one side of the body while the opposite side maintains the upright alignment.

The second half of the first year of development is filled with movements that permit the normal baby to refine this initial contrast between stability and mobility and combine it with a myriad of developmental movements motivated by interest in the environment and the sheer joy of moving.

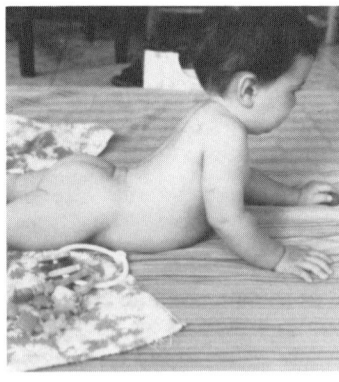

D. Baby extension. Extension in prone at eight months has served to move the center of gravity back toward the pelvis.

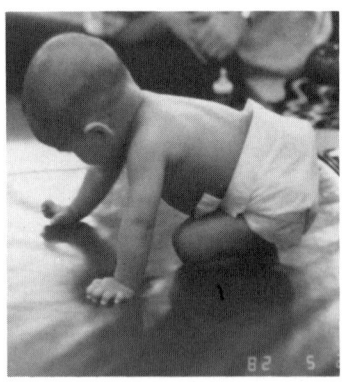

E. Baby flexion. By nine months the baby is moving along the floor in a combination of flexion and extension.

The gradual mastery of flexion, or folding together of the trunk, head and limbs in the supine, or face-up, position, develops parallel to the body extension. Lifting the head often occurs in response to visual stimulus from the adult who stands nearby. It becomes a communication that indicates "I want to come with you" or "I want to be picked up." The infant has previously shown a cessation of postural activity in order to focus the eyes and is now able to move while maintaining visual contact. The intriguing experience of moving feet encourages the baby to reach with the arms and lift the pelvis or the hips to bring the feet closer for visual and tactile examination. This lifting of the lower trunk by the musculature of the ventral surface at this stage of development insures later mobility of the pelvis so essential to sitting and standing. Mobility within the

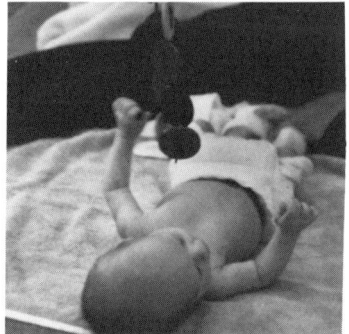
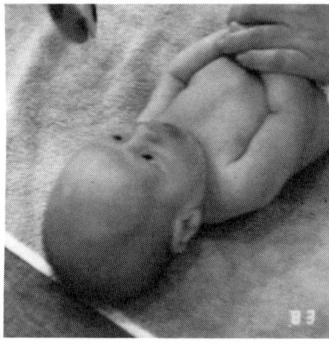

F. Infant stabilizing to direct gaze. This one month old baby tracks the visual stimulus much more readily when her limb movement is controlled for her.

trunk itself prepares the child for the barely perceptible adjustments of position made by an adult who can sit or stand while keeping the eyes focused on an interesting target or while involved in an activity or just lost in thought.

In viewing the dynamic interaction of the visual and postural systems during early development, we can note that the body has developed its extremes of movement in both extension and flexion. At the same time the infant is mastering balance while sitting, which requires a subtle combination of flexion and extension influence, he is also enjoying rocking forward and back on his abdomen. This action often terminates in a sudden landing on the hands and directing of the gaze downward. Especially during the second half of the first year, babies expend great quantities of energy in physical exploration of their environment. They are guided by visual, auditory and tactile novelties and the pleasure of smooth, ever-adapting kinesthetic feedback. The proprioceptive system is clear about its need for change, and the baby openly seeks a new toy or play experience and temporarily rejects the familiar. At this stage one observes a difference in the development of blind infants who cannot rely on visual interest to draw them to further exploration of their surroundings.

The righting and equilibrium reactions that serve to sustain us against gravity have been well described by Karel Bobath, M.D., (1959, 1964) as he studied the absence or partial expression of these reactions in children affected by cerebral palsy, a central nervous system dysfunction. His concepts are helpful in gaining an understanding of the integrative nature of postural stability. Postural reactions form the base for normal movement control and permit predictable relationships to develop between different parts of the body. As the baby masters extension of the body against gravity in the prone position, he is aided by the coordinated antigravity movement of the limbs, as seen in the four-month-old who pulls his elbows back symmetrically to stabilize his shoulders while he rocks to and fro. Due to the head-righting reaction in relation to the trunk, the head position becomes more vertical in relation to the supporting surface. The visual system also seeks an upright alignment from which to view the world, while the vestibular system confirms this useful head position.

The righting or re-positioning of the head in relation to the body position and, conversely, the body in relation to the head, are two of the primary righting reactions that follow lifting the head in relation to the support. These righting responses of the head and body influence all of the baby's early postural changes. The blind child without motor impairment will also show many of these early automatic responses in the adjustment of his posture in space. The blind baby who has his position changed by his caregivers has the opportunity to more effectively use the important cue of proprioceptive experience of the body weight to change the alignment of body parts.

The righting reactions essentially respond to proprioceptive deep-pressure awareness of gravity and are then integrated with the proprioceptive vestibular-based equilibrium reactions. This combination of sensory input gives impulse to the antigravity stability of the trunk, permitting the limbs to move freely. The righting reactions provide central organization and security through the initial deep-pressure proprioceptive experiences. This is the beginning of an interplay between stability and mobility which stays with us throughout life.

In order for the eyes to develop good-quality movement, they also need a stable base which is provided by graded motoric control of the neck in all positions in space. The growing ability of the baby to monitor the position of the head permits more consistent visual examination of interesting objects in the environment. As adults we adapt the head position to meet our visual needs by means of change in the neck alignment. Skilled gymnastic performers must consciously control their automatic reactions in order to accomplish their elaborate flips and turns. Automatically, the head would tend to maintain itself in a position perpendicular to the base or the floor. Dancers must control visual responses by fixing their gaze on a distant point in order to perform a smooth pirouette. The average person pushes his way through a crowd to meet a friend or walks across a footbridge without losing equilibrium by keeping visual contact with his goal and depending on his automatic equilibrium reactions.

During the early months of life when the child lifts his head and moves more in free space, the activity of the vestibular proprioceptive system begins its influence. This is another aspect of the postural reflex mechanism described by Dr. Bobath. (1959, 1964). The vestibular system initially integrates its activity with that of the deep pressure proprioceptors. As the infant is more upright in space, vestibular reactions begin to control the balance, or equilibrium. The equilibrium responses of the human body are automatic and total in nature: the legs and arms move, the trunk curves and the head assumes an alignment related to that of the trunk to shift the center of gravity. All this happens without the central nervous system giving a single conscious command to individual body parts. The maintenance of balance in space is subservient to our conscious behavior.

As the young child still lacks the fluidity of movement necessary to maintain his balance consistently in a coordinated way, he resorts to stepping to avoid a fall. With increased maturity of the postural responses, the trunk will be activated when the balance is threatened, and only in the last moment will protective extension of the limbs be activated.

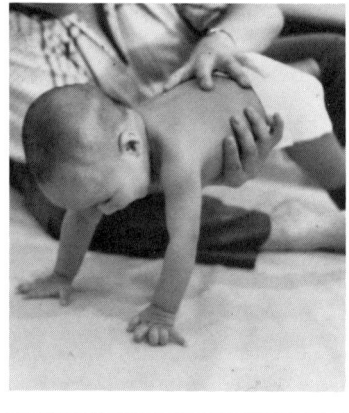

G. Protective extension. Protective extension is one of several automatic responses that reflect the integrity of the postural systems.

The child with marked visual impairment is not able to use the optical righting response to reinforce the head righting that is seen in the Landeau reaction, or extension in prone. The baby who suffers injury to the optic nerve or some other crucial part of the visual system and lacks even general light sensitivity will soon diminish his postural responses and be content with postural adaptations to the immediate surface. Movement responses will be of reduced amplitude and will lack the joy and spontaneity of the normally sighted child. There will tend to be a lack of security and a greater reliance on the righting reactions that depend on deep-pressure proprioceptive information rather than the vestibular proprioceptive reactions. Partial vision or distorted functional vision may create fear of new situations that lack predictability for the child and may reduce significantly the experimentation with postural control that is a part of normal development. The world does not automatically beckon such children to participate. There is no reason for them to maintain balance while striving to reach an object of visual interest. In order to develop a functional postural system, these children need to be given vestibular proprioceptive experiences in play that stimulate their interest in movement and build confidence in their own body. They need to be introduced to the environmental space that they miss through lack of an active visual system.

The postural system is not only useful as a means of dealing with a gravity environment, but also unites with visual responses to create the first communication system known to the infant. The child still being fed in a highchair vehemently turns his head away to indicate that he wants no more dinner. A moment later he points clearly to the plate of his father to request a more interesting menu. Small children are accomplished in managing adults with a mere glance and the simplest of gestures. While this is an interesting and useful development that precedes the organization of the spoken language, it also sets the stage for vision and movement to work together when the schoolchild must copy information from the chalkboard. It reflects the fact that the younger infant has spent much time comparing kinesthetic and tactile feedback with visual feedback to correlate the varied information.

Without an organized postural system, the sensory-motor data acquired by the child from his environment remains fragmented and comparatively disorganized. It lacks a consistent base or frame of

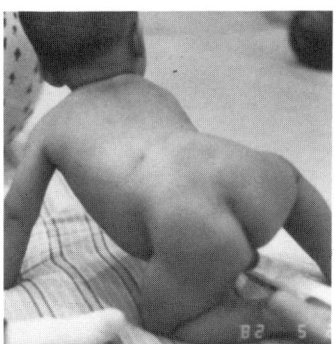 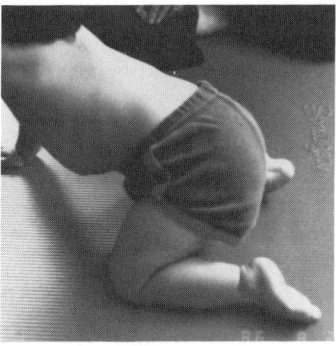

H. Movement on floor. The baby on the left easily shifts to one side to sit. The same transition is an effort for the child on the right because of his wide base of support and poor trunk control.

reference, and compensatory systems tend to come into play to permit functional independence. The problem is seen clearly in children with learning problems who demonstrate postural disorganization. Their central nervous system has never succeeded in relegating postural reactions to the automatic level. Such youngsters are constantly distracted from an immediate task by their need to concentrate on maintaining body balance on the chair or moving themselves across the room. Therapy directed to the organization of postural responses results in positive behavioral changes as well as improved fine coordination. Quality of handwriting control improves, and better organization of school work is noted with no direct practice on the specific task.

Careful observation of a baby's most important first steps reveal that the body responds to the child's visual interest in someone or something across the room or perhaps to the feel of an unexpected shift in the child's center of gravity. Initially, the forward progression is dominated by lateral movement that creates an impression of a toppling forward. As with reaching and other physical activity, the baby does not appear to monitor this forward movement directly, but appears to use a trial-and-error approach followed by self-correction until a more sophisticated movement pattern emerges. Once the baby's system has mastered the ability to walk, the skill is subservient to his interests and his interaction with the environment. Now the possibility exists to explore the visual environment, locate sound sources and match sensory information. The postural and visual systems have developed in a parallel fashion, periodically intertwining their respective contributions into an integrated functional organism.

CHAPTER VII

VISUAL-PERCEPTUAL DEVELOPMENTAL NEEDS OF THE VISUALLY IMPAIRED CHILD

This chapter discusses residual vision as it relates to function and performance. Perception develops in a logical manner. Understanding how visual impairment interferes with this development is of primary importance to the development of a high level of efficiency in residual vision.

Low-Vision Utilization

Low-vision utilization, as stated here, pertains to function and performance within the environment but relates to the definition of vision discussed in a previous chapter. The snare that we often encounter when discussing function is to consider only muscle mechanisms or sensory systems and to relate difficulties in performance solely to isolated problems without considering the interrelationship of sensory, motor, and perceptual processes which stem from a sensory-motor base. For example, the child who is classified as a "toe-walker" is one who walks without touching his heels to the ground. His walking pattern is characterized by short steps with which only the balls of the feet and toes touch the ground and his weight is shifted forward. The common diagnosis based on functional abilities is that the tendons in the back of the legs are too short, causing an inability to extend the legs when walking with a heel-to-toe gait. It is also common to observe that many of these children have emotional difficulties and are usually placed in special education programs.

It has been noted that when specially designed prisms (base-down yoked) are introduced before the eyes of many of these children, the gait is changed from toe-walking to heel-to-toe gaits, and the weight becomes distributed more equally over both feet. The common diagnosis of shortened tendons was based on function and isolated to the supposed inability to extend the heel. This approach does not take into account the profound relationship between sensory and motor processes, particularly the role of vision in performance.

To consider the alternative approach, one must begin by examining behavior as a reflection of the visual process, whether for the sighted or non-sighted individual. When this is done, function and performance become an interaction of physiology, psychological disposition, and the environment, all of which are part of vision and the mainstay of development.

When working with children it is important to realize that the interaction between sensory and motor processes is structured by development. We cannot effectively improve the child's low vision utilization without understanding the developmental level of abilities along with sensory-motor interaction. For this reason, the author has chosen to outline some important considerations of both development and sensory-motor interaction at various ages when attempting to affect low vision utilization. The purpose of any therapy is to reduce the interferences affecting the development and to allow the child to advance at his own rate, not to attempt to make the child advance his development, thereby reducing a manifested developmental lag.

Note: The most effective tools that the optometrist or ophthalmologist has to affect function and performance are the lens and the prism. Unfortunately, the lens and prism have been regarded by many only in their compensatory capacities to correct myopia, hyperopia or astigmatism. The lens and prism have the potential to actually change the relationship of the kinesthetic, proprioceptive, vestibular and other senses to the visual process. When plus lenses or yoked prisms (prisms with the base or thick end in the same orientation before both eyes) are used properly with a person at any age, the use of the ambient and focal process will change, thereby affecting other motor and sensory modalities. Therefore, the clinician who is attempting to provide therapy for a visually impaired or motorically disabled person should not miss the opportunity to work with plus lenses and yoked prisms concurrently with various activities. This idea will be developed further in later chapters. It is emphasized, however, that in all phases of therapeutic treatment, lenses and prisms should be used.

In this chapter various activities designed to affect the developmental nature of the child's vision will be discussed. Appropriate therapeutic lenses and prisms should be used during these activities to reap the full and dynamic effect of this treatment. The activity alone cannot be expected to elicit changes without the proper use of lenses and prisms concurrently. Lenses are usually only used for their effect on the focal aspect of vision. However, lenses and prisms also affect the ambient function relating to motor organization. The young infant or child has a very plastic visual system. Appropriate lenses or prisms can be used effectively to accent relationships between the ambient visual process and the motor system. As the child begins to experience differences in visual and motor relationships, often his performance in other sensory modalities will also be affected.

The First Year
The sight-impaired infant develops rudimentary forms of perception which will form the base for more complex perceptual processes. Since the child's processing abilities are simple during the first year of life, so should be the design of any methods of therapy or stimulation. Overstimulation at any age is as detrimental as understimulation. Overstimulation places demands on the child above his level of abilities. When this happens the child must either push himself beyond his developmental level of abilities or he will show compensating behavior such as avoidance, fatigue or irritability. The long-term result of overstimulation may be physiologic compensation.

Since perception of the figure-ground relationship is the most elementary, and because a child younger than eight-weeks old is primarily developing monocular fixations, an overhead, non-glaring light may be very effective in providing a figure from the background for the child to fixate. The light, being the figure, will elicit a fixation that establishes a figure-ground perception. Of course, the light should not be of an intensity that will cause discomfort to look at directly. Switching the light on and off slowly may also provide variations for perceptual enhancement. Two overhead light sources will permit changes in fixation. They may be constant or slowly alternated. Plus lenses and yoked prisms may be used to provide change to oculomotor and sensory orientation.

Room illumination for the sight-impaired infant should be varied to provide various levels of light stimulation. Lamps should be moved occasionally so that the child experiences light from different directions and so that shadows, which will give added figure-ground dimensions, change in the room. While mobiles are effective in stimulating fixation, they may be overstimulating to many children, causing prolonged fixation on the figure without a release to the ground. It is recommended that mobiles not be used until after eight weeks of age when the child is developing binocular fixation, and then the mobile should be used only for short periods of time.

Since the newborn infant may still be in the tonic neck reflex, focal behavior can be observed on the infant's outstretched hand. This behavior may be enhanced by providing indirect background illumination so that the hand is highlighted as the figure. The opposite method of shining a flashlight directly on the hand in a semi-darkened environment will also provide stimulation for fixation.

Because the newborn is essentially ambient in visual function, tracking movements may be elicited by moving a light or brightly colored object ahead of the child's fixation. Fluorescent objects under ultraviolet and "black" light in a semi-darkened environment may be useful for the sight-impaired child. The ultraviolet light should be positioned not to shine directly at the child's eyes, but on the object being moved. Audible objects (rattles, bells) will also provide good stimulation. All objects should be at close (near-range) distances for the newborn.

The vestibular system is very important to reinforcing eye alignment and direction. Eye movements in response to position change by the mother have been monitored in the unborn infant. From a matching of information received through vision, vestibular, kinesthetic, and proprioceptive stimulation, the infant learns balance and coordinates motor and eye movement skills. Once the infant has achieved binocularity, the information received through vision is no longer segmented and begins to be readily matched with information received through other modalities. However, difficulty in achieving the state of binocularity often occurs because of an inability to utilize various modalities to reinforce visual processing. In turn, processing of information often occurs between isolated senses rather than through multimodality matching.

Moving the child from side to side or rocking the child while the child lies on a large ball will allow vestibular reactions to be matched with vision as the child fixates on a toy. The vestibular stimulation produced will reinforce ocular movements, leading to rudimentary binocular function. The less ability to control focal visual functioning, the more likely it will be to observe shifting eye movements during this activity. It has been noted that strabismic children (particularly exotropes) have demonstrated ocular alignment during these procedures, which have been found useful for children through preschool age. Also, cradling the infant and rocking side to side or varying directions while the infant fixates on the clinician's face will provide visual-vestibular matching of information. Coordinating therapy with neuro-developmental therapy, occupational therapy, and/or physical therapy will be helpful and will provide follow-through.

The focal response when the child is able to accommodate may be further improved by lifting him above the head of the clinician and moving him back and forth from the clinician's face. The infant will enjoy this activity if the clinician talks to him. Turning the child from side to side while this activity is performed will stimulate tracking movements along with convergence and accommodation if he is fixating on the clinician's face.

As focal visual behavior improves, tracking activities should be slowed to allow the child the opportunity to track with fixation. The same objects described previously will be effective in eliciting tracking response. Some creativity on the part of the clinician may generate new and useful objects for this purpose.

The 32-week-old infant, as you will recall, is able to begin to localize objects at greater distances. Activities can be performed by starting at near with visual and audible objects, and backing away while monitoring the infant's fixation and attention. Introducing plus lenses at this time can assist the child in fixating and releasing on near and far objects.

As the infant progresses, the fixation on the object can be stimulated at a distance by making a sound next to a luminous object (i.e., flashlight) and having the infant localize the object auditorily, with visual fixation being the endpoint of the activity.

Note: With all of these activities, the visual abilities of the child will be affected by his particular sight impairment. Working distances that depend on acuity levels and field restrictions must be considered. As this chapter offers suggestions for the individual working with sight-impaired children, it is assumed that refractive considerations have been addressed through a proper clinical examination. The activities may need to be altered for individual children. If the child has a very reduced acuity or field restriction, working distances should be shortened or larger objects used as acuity is lowered. In the case of peripheral field restrictions, smaller objects may be more beneficial than larger ones, or if there is a field restriction impairment on a particular side, the therapist may need to design his activities to approach from the sighted side.

Activities should be designed to enable the child to reinforce vision with motor movement as soon as the child begins to coordinate limb function. Touching, tapping, hitting and pushing movements enable the child to continually match information through vision and its relationship to motor concerning distance, size, shape, form, etc.

When the child is able to crawl, movement should be encouraged. The child may begin to rock back and forth, seeking kinesthetic stimulation. It is not necessary to discourage this. This symptom means the child is not establishing relationships through other modalities to stimulate movement. The therapist must provide reinforcements to develop movement, and once the relationships are established, the rocking behavior will diminish or stop completely. Sounds from several feet away, such as the mother's voice, coupled with visually stimulating objects will develop directionality concepts. By moving one arm of the child forward, an asymmetrical position of balance will be created that may cause the child to shift forward in an attempt to gain back balance. A large ball in front of the child may give the tactual reinforcement. As the child crawls, bumping into the ball will reinforce the concept of direction through touching. If the ball is bright in color (a fluorescent ball under ultraviolet light is effective), it will stimulate visual regard and provide further structure, enabling the child to develop an understanding of the spatial environment.

The Second and Third Year

When the child begins to walk, reinforcement may be needed depending on the impairment. The same techniques used during crawling will be effective. The large ball again will reinforce movement as the child shuffles his feet forward. While crawling and walking the child is relating peripheral central visual and motor processes. The central fixation establishes direction and localization. The peripheral awareness yields organization of field along with concept awareness of space. When these are combined with motor movement, which includes kinesthetic and proprioceptive cues and vestibular cues, the infant reinforces balance and coordination. At all ages, therapy should present the child with situations whereby information may be matched through various motor actions and sensory inputs.

As the child advances, the concept of tri-dimensionality activities should be developed to enable him to manipulate objects by pushing them through holes. It is important to encourage tactual manipulation with visual reinforcement at whatever working distance the child needs to involve vision. Back-lighting to illuminate the hole and/or fluorescent objects enhances the contrast for the sight-impaired child.

Rolling activities will enable the sight-impaired child to maintain much support from the tactual stimulation of being on the floor while exploring body movement initiated from trunk and torso extension. It is important to utilize vision to lead all responses. To accomplish this, it is first necessary to analyze the movements needed to complete a roll. On his back, in order to roll to the right, the child must tuck his chin and turn his head to the right while crossing the left arm over to the right. This will shift the balance to the right. As the child rolls onto his right side, he will need to extend his chin so that the roll onto the stomach will be completed. Once the child is on his stomach, the chin must be tucked and again turned to the right to coordinate a trunk turn in the same direction. A follow-through brings the child onto his back again.

An object that stimulates visual regard may be moved in a way to cause the child to move his head into the desired positions. For example, with the child on his back, if an object is moved to the right and down, causing the child to look down and to the right, the desired chin tuck and head turn to the right will be achieved. As the light is moved out and up, causing the child to have to extend his head to follow it, the extension of the head will be completed, simulating the movements necessary to continue the roll.

Activities should be designed to encourage the child to explore his space world. During this period of development, spatial relationships are being established by matching information about distance between vision and movement. The visually impaired child who has a sight loss will need added reinforcement through other modalities such as audition. An auditory cue coupled with a visual cue provide an understanding of distance when the child matches this information with motor movement.

Visual loss may greatly affect a child's balance, particularly if the loss involves peripheral fields. Peripheral vision provides information concerning location of the self in the environment. A sense of balance is established through the matching of information from vision, vestibular stimulation and kinesthetic information. Since vision is dominant, a loss of this process may impede the child's ability to utilize information from other modalities.

To help the child utilize information, balanced activities that reinforce one another should be assigned to stimulate each of the various modalities. For example, hold the child in your lap while you rock from side to side. As the child moves with you, the vestibular stimulation will be reinforced by the kinesthetic system. By placing a fixed light source in front of the child, the change in location of the light as the child rocks will provide visual reinforcement. Many other techniques and activities may be developed by the creative therapist who understands the need to reinforce information received through more than one modality. Again, lenses and yoked prisms should always be used.

Walking will be enhanced by providing tactual cues for the child. Rails, chairs and tables to hold on to all provide reinforcement. Of course, lighting is extremely important. Too much light is as ineffective as not enough light. Overhead light floods an environment, and shadows are cast beneath the object. Shadows are very important in determining depth relationships. For example, shadows cast by early-morning or late-afternoon sun provide us with information concerning distance of objects because shadows are cast horizontally. Likewise, room lighting that casts shadows to the side of an object will give the child information about depth and his own relationship to objects.

Note: For activities involving visual fixation, the use of a flicker bulb will greatly stimulate visual fixation. A flicker bulb is a special light bulb with an oscillating filament within. When electrified the filament will vibrate at a very rapid rate. Flicker bulbs come in many colors; however, the red bulb has been found most effective in stimulating visual regard. For his protection place a piece of plexiglass between the bulb and the child.

By two-and-one-half years the developmentally mature, sighted child will begin to use himself as a reference point to his environment by relating sound and sight to distances. The sighted child will delight himself by throwing objects around the room and listening to the impact. The developmentally mature, visually impaired child may have difficulty establishing himself as a reference point. Variations in behavior, such as the child holding an object close to his eye to look at it and then holding it in his hand while banging it on the table, would be an indication that the child is reinforcing spatial concepts with tactual and kinesthetic stimulation, but lacks the necessary understanding of space to expand his reference point. This type of behavior would indicate that the child requires greater structure to enable him to explore space. For example, if the child were to throw an object into the distance, the sound of impact may not be related to the action if the child is unable to experience the continuity of space. Having the child first explore the surroundings with motor movement will establish boundaries. The time lapse between the thrown object and sound of impact will now have a motor reference base. Vision can be reinforced further by using highly stimulating, visible objects (i.e., fluorescent balls) coupled with a brief flash of light at the moment of impact coming from the direction of the sound. The child will then use many modalities to develop a concept of space, cause and effect. The simple return of the object by the therapist will help the child establish concept permanence or perceptual constancy. Manipulating it tactually and visually will help the child realize that the object is the same.

Language Development

For the visually impaired child, descriptive concept formation will be difficult because he is unable to visually discern the detailed relationships necessary to establish experience. Because of this, language development may be affected. Language is a symbol code given to some form, object or action. The ability to symbolize occurs when a person perceives some aspect and/or relationship of figure to ground and then presents it by an abstraction. The code of language enables us to relate abstractions to the world that we perceive and vice versa. Being unable to visually discern relationships, an individual will find distorted meanings in abstractions unless he is able to relate the abstraction through another means of sensory-motor exploration and manipulation.

To aid the visually impaired child with language development, it is important to use only concrete descriptive language to help relate and reinforce the child's activities. This does not mean continually barraging the child with verbal patter, but choosing appropriate language to succinctly describe the activity of the child. A simple word that describes what the child is attending to will enable the child to key into the relationship and begin to utilize abstract symbolisms. The development of language will in turn increase the child's ability to further discern relationships visually because it gives the child an abstract dimensionality of experience by which to discern new and more meaningful visual relationships. It has been noted that low plus lenses can greatly improve the child's ability to not only organize visual space and movement, but to reduce visual stress to thereby organize receptive and expressive language.

As the child matures developmentally, spoken language should begin to help him develop new abilities of perceptual transformation (to know how something would look or to understand a thought from another point of view), perceptual constancy (to know how some thing or thought can be the same while allowing for some aspect of change), figure-ground (to hold on to some aspect of detail--either concrete or abstract--allowing all other aspects of perception that develop through sensory-motor exploration). Language can facilitate the perceptual development of the child by giving the child a multifaceted, abstract way to describe and manipulate his experiences.

The concept development of a ball for a visually impaired child may proceed by the child first visualizing a circular disk. A new dimension may be experienced when the child manipulates it by touch and feels the round nature of the ball. By reinforcing the word "ball" with the description "round," the therapist has given abstract meaning in concrete terms to the child's visual and tactual-motor experience. New perceptual dimensionality may be added when the child is given two balls, one large and the other small. As the child perceives the similarities and differences of the balls, perceptual constancy is developed, i.e., when the child holds on to one aspect (the roundness) but allows for change (the size). At appropriate moments, the words "large ball" and "small ball" develop symbols to relate to the concrete perceived qualities. What the ball looks and feels like as it is rotated in his hands helps develop the child's concurrent transformational perceptions.

The older child will eventually use language to describe and reinforce his perception of the environment and provide a new structural dimension to vision in perceiving new relationships. By three-and-one-half to four years of age the visually impaired child should begin to use abstract symbols to develop new dimensions of other symbols. For example, the child may not have the ball available but should be able to describe it as being "round and big" and, when asked through language how else a ball might look, would say "round and small" or "red" or "it rolls." It is not the purpose of this chapter to describe the relationship between language and visual development for all stages. Rather, it is intended to point out that language, through representative coding, is related to the child's development of visual-perceptual skills and experiences, and that the therapist can and should consider the use of appropriate language in program development as a tool to enhance vision and perception.

The Fourth and Fifth Years

Depending on the amount and type of sight loss and visual abilities, many visually impaired four- and five-year-old children will show marked difficulties with perceptual-motor activities. Since vision for these children is unstable and lacking experience, difficulties will be observed with movement and coordination. To improve the difficulties the visually impaired child has with educating his residual vision to lead motor movement and conceptualize space, therapy must be structured to work at the child's level of ability by presenting activities that permit him to explore without fear.

Movement that explores body position in space is an essential component for spatial concept formation. Leading the child into various positions, beginning with the child on his stomach or back, enables him to experience kinesthetic and proprioceptive reinforcement of body position. Initially, he may avoid visual fixation on his own body movement. When the child experiences the feeling of raising a foot or an arm with the help of a therapist, the child should be encouraged to fixate on the elevated arm or leg. A game may be played where the therapist raises or extends an arm or a leg of the blindfolded child, and the child must somehow describe or point with another arm where the appendage is. As the child succeeds in understanding body movement through feeling, visual fixation can be added by having the child find the elevated or raised appendage visually and reach out with another arm or hand to touch it while fixating on it.

The next step would be to raise the child to a crawling position. Fixation on the fluorescent-colored backs of his hands will be stimulated by overhead ultraviolet light. Using a different color on each hand will allow color differentiation and controlled fixation to auditory commands. Front and backward directionality concepts can be explored also. The child can explore balance by raising an arm or leg. Balance occurs when the child develops the ability to counterbalance movement. The motor equivalent movement enables the child to develop stability and coordination. Without the reactive movement, balance is lost.

Progressing to kneeling and finally to standing allows the child to explore new situations from a safe plane of reference. Movement while standing should proceed from first feeling to being coupled with vision. The reason for this progression is that many children (sighted and sight-impaired) will often, in their attempt to utilize vision, suppress or suspend information received from motor movement.

At this age it is important to develop projectionality and concepts of direction. In other words, visual space and visual projections do not or should not change when the child closes his eyes. Visual projection should merely be transferred to kinesthetic reinforcement. For example, a child who looks at a ball 10 feet in front of him lines himself up with the ball and proceeds to walk to it. If the child were to be blindfolded after becoming visually oriented, the child would have to rely on feeling motor movement (the kinesthetic and proprioceptive systems) to be able to direct himself correctly.

Seventh, Eighth and Ninth Years

Depending on the visual impairment and how development has been affected, a wide range of behaviors may be observed in the child. The child whose impairment has not interfered with his progress will be ready to learn perceptual skills and should be worked with in a variety of ways. The child whose impairment has interfered with his progress may be delayed several years. To attempt to introduce higher order perceptual skills to this child would push him beyond his level of perceptual abilities. Frustration will be experienced by both child and therapist, for progress will be very slow.

It is necessary, therefore, to observe the child's behaviors, to know the child through how he acts. If the child is still displaying behaviors and needs of a four-year-old, then habilitation programming should be organized accordingly. This chapter is not meant to be a "cookbook" for designing habilitation programs for the low vision child, but to impart to the reader the developmental needs of the visually impaired child. If those needs are met appropriately, habilitation will proceed in a natural manner with a minimum of frustration and trauma to both the child and the therapist.

The seventh, eighth and ninth years are important in developing higher level visual-perceptual abilities in the low vision child. This doesn't mean that visual-motor activities should be discontinued. Rather, the approach should include a variety of activities.

Visual tracking activities should be continued. Flashlight tracking games will stimulate interest, and since projection concepts should be developing at this stage (by six years developmentally), the child should be able to perform them. For example, the author has developed a game called "Star Wars." Six large fluorescent numbers (bases one through six) are hung on a wall in two columns. An ultraviolet light suspended from the ceiling will illuminate the numbers if the room lights are dimmed. The child holds one flashlight with a colored filter (red) and the therapist another with a different colored filter (green). The different colors will enable the child to identify his own light. Using some imagination, the child's light may represent a popular hero from a science fiction fantasy and the therapist's light, of course, a villain. The child should shine his light on base number one and proceed to base two, three, four and so on. The therapist's light should move with the child's light. The object of the game is for the child to move his light to each of the bases in sequence without being tagged by the therapist's light when the child is off the base. After two successive tags, the positions are reversed.

This activity develops tracking skills through fixation on the light, but more importantly, it develops a relationship between peripheral and central vision. The base and the therapist's light will both be in the periphery when the child fixates on his own light. One reason for success in moving the light from one base to another without being tagged will occur when the child can relate his peripheral vision with central vision. The low vision child often has difficulty in using both together. Peripheral and/or central field losses do not mean that the child will be unable to perform this type of activity. However, the visual process must be worked with in order to develop the necessary skills.

As with children without sight impairments, often a child will concentrate so intently on one aspect of vision that he may not process important information from another aspect of vision. For example, the child engrossed in watching a bicyclist go by may trip over the rock that lies in his path. Relating peripheral vision to central vision is important to developing timing, coordination and balance. Perceptually, the peripheral field is the ground to fixation and should relate constancy through which the individual can compare size, distance and motion to other sensory-motor functions to develop an understanding of space volume. When there is a mismatch of information, understanding of the relationship between space and time is distorted. This is usually an unconscious distortion. For example, the person who swings the bat too early or too late at a pitched ball may actually perceive the ball to be at another location than it is.

Walking rail activities (walking on a board placed on the floor) while fixating on an object ahead is good for developing visual and kinesthetic awareness. A metronome beat for each step can be incorporated.

Strip fixations will also help develop visual efficiency between peripheral and central vision. Two strips of letters are mounted on the wall approximately two-and-one-half feet apart. The child should stand four to five feet from the letters and proceed to read a letter from each column, starting first with the top left letter, then to the top right letter, and so on. The quick eye movements that are made when looking from one letter to another are a motor match of information received from peripheral and central vision concerning direction and distance. Losing one's place will indicate inappropriate sensory-motor matching and/or suspension of information. Also, a metronome beat can add rhythm as progress is achieved. Lenses and prisms provide a means to directly affect vision, timing, and spatial concepts during these activities.

Developing visual imagery and memory is important at this stage of development. Through visualization, problem solving and thought processing continue to develop. Recognizing part and whole relationships are an important part of visualization and memory. Activities should be used to develop these skills. For example, blocks may be organized in a design. The child is to explore the design through visual and tactual-kinesthetic means and then reconstruct it with other blocks from memory. Perceptual transformation and constancy skills can be worked with by asking the child to construct the design as if he were sitting on the other side of the table. The child will have to visualize the design and transpose it in his mind. A child who is having difficulty with laterality (knowing his left from his right) will have difficulty with transformations because perceptual constancy has not been established. The child cannot perceive a difference between an orientation of blocks one way or the other. Color coding the table and the child's hands may help. For example, a piece of red tape on the right hand and green tape on the left hand will help to visually reinforce the laterality concept.

To develop laterality skills, other activities may be performed using red and green tape on the child's hands and feet (red on the right). Activities such as "Simon Says" can require matching the right and left hand to auditory commands. Directionality concepts (projecting left and right into the field) can be developed through visual cues from the leader of "Simon Says." To determine a correct movement, the red or green tape on the child and the therapist should be matched.

Another visual memory activity that is effective in building laterality, directionality and imagery skills is to play tic-tac-toe from memory (without writing down the moves). This will be a challenge for both the child and the therapist.

Activities such as these will help the child develop skills of visual processing that will improve his efficiency and organization of thought and problem solving. The therapist who understands some of the basics behind the visual and perceptual processes can develop activities pertinent to the needs of the low vision child.

The reader may question what feeling, kinesthetic movement, spatial relationships, and other perceptual developments have to do with getting the child to see and use optical aids. The following section is devoted to explaining these relationships.

The Use of Optical Aids
Visually impaired children usually do not respond successfully to optical aids until at least three years of age (developmental age). It takes that long for a child to develop the perceptual skills necessary to understand visual space through the impairment that he has. If a telescope or magnifier which further distorts space is placed before

the child's eyes, matching of information from other sensory modalities is greatly hindered. By three years of age those children who have exceptional perceptual skills should be able to adapt to some simple forms of near magnification. There is no magic age. It depends on the child's visual-perceptual flexibilities and, most importantly, his ability to match information.

As mentioned previously, it is very important to detect the visual impairment as early as possible. A visual examination by a qualified optometrist or ophthalmologist within the first four weeks after the child is born is recommended. If an impairment is diagnosed, medical and low vision treatment and a habilitation program may be developed to meet the child's present and future needs. In the case of planning for low vision services, the optometrist, parents and other involved professionals should discuss the child's potential future needs for optical aids. They need to decide what can be done to develop the necessary perceptual skills to use the optical aid(s) prior to the prescription of the aid(s). An interdisciplinary approach including therapy will make the introduction of optical aid(s) less demanding and stressful on the child.

Although the type of therapy designed to prepare the child to use optical aids may vary considerably, depending on the child's developmental age, physical abilities, perceptual abilities, intelligence and environmental surroundings, a basic understanding of the optics of the aid, how space is distorted through the aid, and, most importantly, what perceptual skills are needed to reinforce successful use of the aid will enable the therapist to design a program to meet the child's needs. The following procedures are basic functional processes involved in utilizing optical aids successfully. These techniques have been developed through an understanding of the perceptual skills involving organization of field and the interactions between the various sensory-motor functions. The therapist, through creative thinking and understanding the basic functional processes involved, should be able to adapt these techniques to the developmental needs of the child and his environment.

Telescopic aids vary greatly in magnification and field of view. They also differ in size and type (e.g., hand-held, head-borne, spectacle-mounted). Since all telescopes (except for a reverse telescope) distort space by magnifying the object, reducing the field of view, and projecting the image of the object closer, many children and adults will become greatly disoriented initially. The disorientation occurs because the sensory information received through the eye from the optical aid has not been matched or has been inappropriately matched with information received through other sensory-motor feedback systems. Experience has not been supportive to enable the person to adapt to a new spatial construct. For example, the reduction of the field of view and magnification cause the person to view a relatively small island in the environment. The peripheral vision that is now sacrificed was important to the person for establishing a total organization of field or a part-to-whole concept. The peripheral vision helped to reinforce balance as well as develop an understanding of time and distance relationships.

Initially, the child may hold the telescope before his eye to look through it but not know at what or where he is looking. If the child is standing, he will often begin to wobble because of loss of balance. Sometimes this initial disorienting experience can be a negative one despite all the hard work and good intentions of the optometrist and parents to give the child an optical aid. The failure in use of the optical aid and the negative experience may be avoided by some preliminary work with the child. The developmental activities described earlier are important to stimulate and develop sensory-motor processing. They should be performed regardless of whether or not optical aids are to be used.

If a telescope is to be prescribed for a child, the parent, educator, or other therapist might engage in some game-like activities to develop some of the specific skills needed. Spatial direction and projection are developmentally established through motor reinforcement. Therefore, the maintenance of motor and kinesthetic feedback are extremely important for success with optical aids. Kinesthetic awareness coupled with tactual and auditory stimulation will enable the child to maintain organization of the spatial environment. The first procedure (Stage One) to stimulate this process is the for child to close his eyes and reach out and grasp a pencil that the optometrist is holding. The child is then told that the optometrist is going to move the pencil. The object of the activity is to see if he can keep his head pointed directly at the pencil. As the pencil is moved, the child will be aware of the position of the pencil by kinesthetic reinforcement through his extended arm. Success in head orientation to the position of the pencil is the goal of this procedure.

Stage Two repeats the procedure, but this time instruct the child to hold his head still and follow the pencil only with his closed eyes. At some point after the pencil has been stopped the optometrist should say "open your eyes," and success would be rated on how close the child's eyes are to the pencil. Once the child can maintain the appropriate direction in relation to the moving pencil through kinesthetic reinforcement from the extended arm, the next procedure should be tried.

Stage Three uses auditory and kinesthetic reinforcement of visual direction. A bell is used instead of a pencil. The child holds the bell and Stages One and Two should be performed again for transitional purposes. After the child has adapted to the sound of the bell, remove the child's hand and ask him to point to the bell, first with head movement and then eye movement. (Remember, the eyes should be closed during the procedures and should only be opened as reinforcement to the child.) Successful orientation to the direction and position of the bell indicates that the child is utilizing audition to reinforce the kinesthetic position sense.

In Stage Four the bell is moved farther and farther from the child to determine if directional concepts can still be maintained. Variations in these procedures should be performed by having the child stand and balance on one foot, rather than being seated. As success is achieved, the child may be turned around and around in the center of the room with his eyes closed. He is instructed to stop turning, face, and point in the direction of the bell.

The older (eight to nine years developmentally) may enjoy playing the game "North, South, East and West." The child stands in the center of the room and memorizes the direction of each wall marked North, South, East and West. When the child closes his eyes the optometrist asks the child to point to the wall that is called out. If the child correctly points to all of the walls, turn him 180 degrees (face him opposite the original direction) and repeat the procedure. A 90-degree change in direction, turning the child around and around, and then stopping will require the child to rely on kinesthetic movement to maintain spatial orientation.

Several days, weeks, or even months of repeating these procedures, and other similar procedures, may be necessary before an optical aid should even be tried. When success is achieved with these activities, similar therapy with the telescope itself can begin.

Begin using the telescope in the same manner described in Stage One, only have the child hold the telescope to one of his closed eyes while reaching out and holding the pencil with the other hand. Do the procedure. Since the pencil will be too close for the child to view it through the telescope, the idea is to simply set up a procedure that causes the child to continue utilizing the kinesthetic and vestibular systems to reinforce directional concepts. Most importantly, it is success oriented because the demands are within the level of the perceptual abilities of the child.

Proceed to auditory stimulation at a near range, still not requiring the child to find the bell visually but requiring the child to key off of auditory sounds to reinforce kinesthetic directional awareness. With success, remove the bell to a distance farther away, as outlined in Stage Four. Success is not measured on finding the bell visually through the telescope, but only on directional orientation.

When directional orientation is achieved, the child should be asked what he sees. The child may have difficulty describing what he sees because of the lack of experience in understanding things through magnification.

The therapist may attempt to help bring the child's fixation through the telescope to the desired position by flashing a light or making a movement to enable the child to see some change in contrast and figure-ground relationship. Changing fixation from one point to another at distance should be the next step. Auditory stimulation at the fixation point together with pointing first in the direction of the sound should precede attempting to locate the object visually.

Conclusion

Kinesthetic and auditory reinforcement is very important in establishing and maintaining spatial direction and perception. The child who does not succeed in using telescopic aid prescriptions fails because he is unable to maintain an organization of space through reinforcement from sensory-motor processing. By practicing these procedures daily and encouraging and reinforcing the child's responses, the optometrist will be developing the basic functional processes necessary for utilizing the optical aid which will maximize the child's vision.

Training for Utilization of Near Optical Aids

The great variation between the types of near optical aids (i.e., stand magnifiers, hand-held magnifiers, spectacle-mounted binoculars, and monoculars makes one general approach for therapy difficult. This section will be concerned only with the basic functional processes needed to use the aid.

Since the near optical aid distorts space through magnification and reduces the field of view, it brings the projection of an image closer, and disorientation may occur with the child or adult for the same reasons as occur with telescopic aids. The type of disorientation, however, will be in loss of place in near space. Since near optical aids are used mainly for reading, indications of difficulty using the aid may appear as behavioral symptoms. For example, the child may experience loss of place, have difficulty understanding what he is reading, or have difficulty remembering what he has read.

If a near optical aid is to be prescribed, several procedures may be effective in developing the appropriate perceptual skills needed to use the aid prior to its prescription. For all near optical aid use, tactile-kinesthetic reinforcement is important to maintain spatial organization of the field. When this is lost, disorientation occurs and the person will have difficulty knowing where he is looking. The procedure to begin with is touching, understanding direction through kinesthesia, and then looking through the aid.

Utilizing this approach, the therapist may begin by having the child reach with his hand into a sandbox or onto a table and find an object (block, marble, etc.) by feeling for it. (Having the child close his eyes initially may make the procedure more effective.) Once the child has found the object tactually, have the child do whatever he has to in order to see it. The child may have to bring the object very close. A variation of this activity would be to play the game "What Is It?" Several different but familiar objects should be placed in the child's field. When the child finds one, he must determine what it is only by feeling it. After guessing what it is, the child may then look at it to determine if he is right. At this time the therapist should reinforce the child's decision, and if the guess was incorrect, the therapist should help the child determine what it is, preferably by describing salient features of the object in order to have the child finally determine the correct answer.

These are preliminary activities designed to stimulate tactual and kinesthetic awareness. Both of these processes will be used to reinforce visual organization of the field. This can be accomplished by having the child hold a cardboard tube or a large piece of cardboard with a hole in the center up to one eye (the other eye should be occluded). The tube should touch the eye. With the other hand the child should hold a peg, light or small object. The child should be told to be aware of feeling the object and then to find the object while looking through the tube. The purpose of the tactual and kinesthetic stimulation is to reinforce the child's visual organization of the field, thereby enabling the child to "feel" the correct direction before sighting through the tube. Auditory stimulation can also be added to give another dimension to the directional stimulation. Once the child has sighted the object through the tube, have him move the tube toward the object, while still sighting through the tube, until the tube slides over the object. During this step the child should continue to hold the object with the other hand for added reinforcement. This procedure will develop sighting ability while reinforcing vision with tactile and kinesthetic cues.

The following procedures for varying types of near optical aids, utilize tactual and kinesthetic reinforcement of vision. These procedures may be adapted to the specific instructions of the aid or the child's special needs. It is important that appropriate lighting be used.

Hand-Held Magnifiers
Since the variation of power of the magnifier will require specific working distances, the reader should refer to chapter 10 to learn how to determine the appropriate working distance. Once this is calculated, the therapist or the examining clinician will be able to organize the activity so that the appropriate working distance for the magnifier is the end result.

In the procedure previously described, the hand-magnifier may be substituted for the tube. The child should touch the object with one hand and hold the magnifier up to touch the unoccluded eye. Since the power of lens will initially not be at the appropriate working distance, the object will be blurred and out of focus. This is desirable because the child must now key into his tactual and kinesthetic cues to learn where the object is. The child should then, in a similar manner to using the tube, move the magnifier toward the object until the object is clear and the appropriate working distance has been verified. Variations of this activity would be to hold the magnifier on the object being held with the other hand and move the magnifier up toward the eye until the object is in focus. The therapist will have to work with the child to determine where the child's head should be positioned for best viewing.

The proper distance to hold the magnifier from the object is learned through kinesthetic reinforcement to vision. The sense of feeling and knowing the location of the arm and hand that is holding the magnifier develops the understanding of where the magnifier is to be positioned. If the child has continuous difficulty learning where to position the magnifier, the therapist may want to work in some other auditory-tactual- kinesthetic awareness activities involving distance determination. For example, with the child's eyes closed the therapist should hold a dowel or peg at different distances in front of the child. A bell rung near the dowel will give some directional awareness. The child should reach out and find the dowel with one hand and with the other hand place rings or circular objects over the dowel. Varying the distance of the dowel will stimulate the kinesthetic awareness of different distances.

As the child becomes proficient in focusing the aid, and the therapist begins to advance the child with the magnifier to other activities, the child will proceed more rapidly if the therapist keeps the importance of tactual-kinesthetic reinforcement to visual organization in mind. By having the child simply touch or point to what he is attempting to magnify, the child will be more aware of where in his visual field he is directing the magnifier.

Stand Magnifiers

Since stand magnifiers have their working distances already set by their structure, the therapist need only be concerned with getting the child to place it in the correct location on the page. This may be accomplished by first having the child feel the page and finding the upper-left corner both visually and tactually. The magnifier should be brought to the upper-left corner on the page and then moved down until the first print is observed. Depending on the type of stand magnifier, it can slide across the line, allowing the child to read the words through the magnifier. It is important that the child mark the beginning of the line with his finger. Again, this gives the child tactile and kinesthetic knowledge of what line he is on. When the child gets to the end of the line, he only has to move the magnifier back to the finger and drop one line on the page to be positioned at the next line.

Headborne Magnifiers

These may include clip-on magnifiers, bifocals, reading lenses in glasses, or any microscopic aid that has a limited working distance. These will be more appropriate for older children (eight and above) because of the coordination needed. A younger child with superior perceptual skills may adapt with some training. These aids require that whatever is viewed be placed close to the aid. The therapist should be familiar with the specific instructions for use of the particular aid and then adapt tactile and kinesthetic cues to enable the child to understand distance relationships needed to focus the aid.

Focusing the aid on the child's hand is a good way to begin. As the child's hand comes into focus, an object or print on paper can be inserted into his hand. This process may be done along with some of the preliminary distance-judging activities described earlier.

Reading sentences may offer more difficulty since the distance will change and the print will be out of focus if the child turns his head. An effective activity in developing this technique involves making a device with an ordinary coat hanger. Bend the wire so that it fits over and around the crown of the child's head. On either side of the forehead attach two pencils that project forward the exact distance of the focal length of the lens (i.e., if a +10 D lens is used, then the 10-cm focal length of the lens would require the pencils to also be 10 cm long). When the child holds the paper in front of his face to read, have him move the paper back and forth. The pencils will keep the paper always at the correct working distance.

Telemicroscopes

These are spectacle-mounted microscopic devices designed to have fixed working distances beyond the characteristic working distance of the dioptic value. The child will have to sight through the aid while keeping the printed material at a specified working distance. These sophisticated devices are usually prescribed for purposes such as reading or working with chemicals that should not be brought close to the face.

Since head positioning is very important for using these aids successfully, some of the activities described earlier may be effective for preliminary training. Another activity that has been found effective is to mount a light on the child's head. (Headlamps with a light attached to an elastic strap are sold at most hardware or sporting goods stores at a minimal cost.) The child should first touch the page to gain tactile and kinesthetic reinforcement, and then move his head so that the light shines on the page. When the telemicroscope is positioned before the child's eye(s), the procedure should be the same--touch first and then align the light. When the light shines on the finger touching the page, the child has only to move himself closer to or farther from the page to position the aid at the correct focal length.

If a typoscope (a black marker with a slit in it that is placed over the reading material) is used to help the child find his place, it should not be used in place of pointing to and touching the page. Pointing and touching give the child multi-sensory- motor experiences that reinforce vision. If the typoscope is used, have the child point at the same time.

CHAPTER VIII

LOW-VISION SERVICE DELIVERY SYSTEM AND ITS FUTURE

Historically, low vision services have developed from a concept that optical aid dispensing by an optometrist or optician included only simple types of devices such as hand-held magnifiers in very limited powers. Over the past 50 years, low- vision services have expanded to include the services of many professionals who serve the unique and individual needs of the visually impaired person. In addition, the optical aids have become more sophisticated and enable the practitioner to be more selective in meeting the needs of the individual. The present concept recognizes that the needs of the visually impaired person cannot be met by one professional alone. A multidisciplinary approach has evolved as the most effective way of rehabilitating the individual. The multidisciplinary philosophy emphasizes that improvement in performance is not a function of increased ability to see clearly, i.e., improvement in visual acuity. This philosophy maintains that the improvement in acuity is only one factor. Very often, improvement in acuity alone is not sufficient to improve the performance of the individual.

The low vision service is defined as "a professional environment in which assessment, and prescriptive, instructive, and/or rehabilitative activities are provided for the visually impaired person, either directly or by referral." The service includes any and all professionals devoted to serving the needs of the visually impaired. It differs from a low vision evaluation in that the evaluation is part of the service. The low vision clinical analysis and evaluation involves the judgment of function and analysis of performance.

In order to accurately determine the abilities through clinical analysis and evaluation, it becomes necessary to analyze the person's abilities from different professional perspectives. The low vision examination that is performed by the optometrist or ophthalmologist may be able to determine certain aspects of limitation of the individual. However, the capabilities seen from this perspective alone may not identify the complete potential of the individual. It becomes necessary to incorporate functional analysis by other disciplines or professionals to complement those measurements taken in the vision examination. It is necessary to not only perform a clinical analysis and evaluation, but also to perform a low vision functional assessment involving a behavioral assessment of the visually impaired person to determine the historical background of the person that will influence function and performance. The historical background includes psycho-physical abilities and socioeconomic and cultural influences of the goals, interests and expectations of the person.

Once the assessment is performed and information about the functional abilities of the individual is combined with information determined from the clinical analysis and evaluation, a more complete picture of the abilities and needs of the individual can be made. When all of this is compiled, then a service model is functioning. The prescription of optical aids can be determined not simply based on an acuity measurement, but upon the functional abilities of the individual. It may also be necessary to develop training and instructional programs for the individual to improve his ability to utilize the optical aids in various environmental settings. These training or instructional activities for the visually impaired person are designed to cause positive behavioral changes, thereby reducing the handicap and improving performance. These training and instructional activities can and should be developed on all levels of service. This means that the patient should receive adequate training and instruction in the use of the optical aids from the prescribing practitioner. In addition, special perceptional training programs may be developed to improve the function of vision prior to or after prescription.

Continuation of instructional activities can and should be delivered by rehabilitative professionals and educators in environmental settings that offer varying demands. Any difficulties encountered through the use of the optical aids can be remedied by referral back to the appropriate professional and/or by changing the instructional program. It is imperative that periodic performance evaluations be conducted in order to determine if there are any changes in the individual's use of his vision. Due to the dynamic nature of the visual impairment, periodic evaluations of the patient should occur to ensure that the examination assessment and instruction program meets the rehabilitative needs of the patient and the low vision service. Although development of low vision services may be extremely important, there are certain limitations from both within and outside the field of vision impairment and blindness.

To the general public, the term "blind" means total loss of vision. This causes much difficulty because the general public does not differentiate between a partial loss of vision and total blindness. Also, the visually impaired person tends to avoid low vision clinics that are in rehabilitation/blindness agencies because of their association with the term blind. There are many reasons for maintaining the word blind in agency titles and for the development of legislation; however, the reasons are extraneous to the issue at hand. The inclusion of the word blind in low vision services has actually limited the extent to which the services have been effective for dealing with the needs of the total population.

Outside the field of vision impairment and blindness, there remain barriers to the development of low vision services primarily because the public and other professionals are largely unaware of the concept of low vision service. Unfortunately, there are still many doctors who will not refer the visually impaired individual to a low vision service because they do not understand this concept. The feeling is that a person with visual impairment, whether it is central vision loss or peripheral vision loss, is blind and that nothing more can be done. The result is that individuals with usable vision, although visually impaired, are forced to accept blindness rehabilitation instead of rehabilitation through low vision services. The consumer, unaware that low vision services are available, spends many years searching for a cure without success, only to be forced into a blindness system. The problem also remains that even within the blindness and visually impaired field, there are many professionals who do not refer visually impaired individuals for rehabilitative low vision services for reasons similar to those mentioned above.

There is a wide range of optical aids, electronic aids and non-optical aids that can benefit the consumer. Technological advancement of new types of optical aids, however, has essentially come to a halt. Yet, by the year 2000 it is predicted that the population of those who are visually impaired and over the age of sixty in the United States will at least double. Because age is the greatest predictor of vision impairment, and there is an expected population increase in those over 65 years of age, this statistic could increase substantially. In addition, because of medical and surgical advances, fewer individuals will go totally blind, but a greater percentage of population will become visually impaired.

Recognizing what is essentially on our doorstep, private industry has voiced an interest in attempting to develop new and improved low vision devices. Much of the industry, however, has stalled in making the first step because of the lack of marketing demand at this time. By marketing demand, we mean consumers who will purchase the products. Since the majority of visually impaired persons are not referred to low vision services, the demand does not reflect the actual consumer need. Many private industries are unwilling at this time to put substantial amounts of money into research and development of new types of optical aids.

There are other complicating factors impeding the development of complete low vision services. All rehabilitative services are expensive, and at this time most of these costs are covered by the visually impaired person. This is because there are no overall legislative mechanisms to cover low vision services for the majority of visually impaired individuals. Presently, low vision services are provided under four basic legislative programs. These are the Social Security Act, the Education of the Handicapped Act, the Rehabilitation Act, and the Veterans and Uniforms Services Benefits. These four programs cover only a small portion of the total number of visually impaired individuals in the United States.

Briefly, the Social Security Act, or Title 20, was passed by Congress in 1975 as Public Law #93-647 as an amendment to the Social Security Amendment of 1974. It provides funds allocated to states, on a population basis, by the federal government and requires no additional funds by state or employers. Presently, there are only 13 states that directly target Title 20 moneys to services for the blind and visually impaired. Other states provide services to the blind as a component of various other service definitions. Analysis of service descriptions shows that the money from this law is used in training motor and mobility skills, personal care, home management, and communication skills and arranging for the provision of aids, supplies and appliances. Precedent has been set in New York and Virginia for reimbursement of low vision services through Title 20 when not covered by Medicare and Medicaid. To qualify for Title 20, a person must be over the age of 65.

Title 19 (Grants to States for Medical Assistance Programs) is also known as Medicaid. The Medicaid program was enacted in 1965 as an amendment to the Social Security Act. It is also the largest government health-care program. Medicaid is a federal- state agreement. This means that federal moneys are allocated for medical needs only if the state will match moneys for the same purpose. It is difficult to determine whether low vision services are provided through Medicaid in all states. The qualified person must receive in-patient hospital care, out-patient hospital care, rural health-clinic service, other laboratory and X-ray services, skilled nurses facility services, in-home health care for individuals 21 years and older, early periodic screening, diagnosis and treatment for individuals under 21 years, and family planning and physician services. By simply reading the statutes for Medicaid, it seems there is a greater potential for low vision services. Individual contact for state agencies, however, has found that money through Title 19 varies from state to state. Questions pertaining to the use of Medicaid money should be referred directly to the individual state Medicaid agency.

Title 18 (Health Insurance for Aged and Disabled) is Medicare. Section 1843 of Title 18 of the Social Security Act establishes additional health coverage for people aged 65 and over. Some people under 65 or disabled are receiving benefits under Title 16 (Grants to States for the Aged, Blind, and Disabled or for Such Aid and Medical Assistance for the Aged--FSI) or Title 4 (Grants to States for Aid and Services to Needy Families with Children and Child Welfare Services--AFDC). Unlike Medicaid, Medicare does not require matching funds by the state. Medicare does not officially cover low vision services, but a limited telephone survey (unpublished survey conducted by the author in 1982) found that there are some clinics receiving reimbursement for low vision services and others for optical aids. It was discovered that these clinics are hospital based. Possible reasons for this inconsistency may be variations in interpretation by insurance intermediaries and/or the classification of services based on medical treatment other than low vision services.

Title 5 (Maternal and Child Health and Crippled Children Services Act) is intended to increase services in rural and economically distressed areas. Low-vision services may be reimbursed except when such services are performed in a clinic or other institution. Low-vision services require prior authorization.

Title 2 (Federal Old Age Survivors and Disability Insurance--CASDI) enables disabled persons to qualify through the state agency administering the plan approved under the Vocational Rehabilitation Act. Qualified clients may receive both low vision services and follow-up low vision care during vocational rehabilitation. Similar to Title 2, Title 4 (AFDC) provides low vision services for disabled individuals for vocational rehabilitation.

The second major program is Public Law 94-142 (Education for All Handicapped Children Act of 1975). Its purpose is to provide appropriate education for all children and to alter programs when needed to meet a child's unique needs. This law emphasizes the individualized education program, i.e., through special education in related services. P.L. 94-142 provides low vision care in addition to speech pathology, audiology, psychological services, physical and occupational therapy, recreation, and medical and counseling services. Problems have occurred in various communities with regard to delivering learning-disability programs to visually impaired children (Padula 1979). It appears that, due to either misinterpretation of the law itself or a lack of understanding of the development of learning disability, learning disability in some children is being diagnosed as being caused primarily by physical handicap. In turn, services are developed and provided only to affect the handicap, i.e., an optical aid or a hearing aid will be given to the child in order to improve the sight or hearing. The problem is that there is no way to directly correlate the learning disability with the physical handicap; therefore, many children who should be receiving learning-disability programs in addition to the optical and/or hearing aids may not be receiving the appropriate services.

The third important program is the Rehabilitation Act of 1973. This law provides services or aids to the handicapped to render the handicapped person employable. Congress has not included this section in appropriations. Under Section 721, funding is designated to states to provide independent-living services to older blind individuals. Low-vision is included in this area.

The Veterans in Uniform Services benefits provides low vision services, optical aids, and training in the use of aids for legally blind veterans. If not legally blind, they are entitled to receive in- and outpatient medical treatment for their disability. This treatment can include low vision care. Under the Veterans in Uniform Services Benefit, CHAMPUS may include low vision examinations but will not pay for low vision aids. Training in the use of these aids is included as a total rehabilitation package. CHAMPUSVA, a cost-sharing extension of CHAMPUS, extends the coverage and includes some low vision services to children of totally and permanently disabled veterans and children of veterans who died of service-connected causes. Usually, the child must be under 18 years of age, although those incapable of self-support because of mental or physical incapacity that existed before age 18 may be eligible indefinitely.

These four basic legislative mechanisms offer limited reimbursement for low vision service. Fortunately, private insurance companies are beginning to recognize the needs of visually impaired individuals, and some insurance companies are including low vision services in their coverage. These insurance companies are limited. Very often, even if the company has set a policy to offer low vision services, it is misinterpreted by employees and requires repeated and persistent contact with and explanation by the policy holder and the servicing doctor.

The Future of Low-Vision Services

Although legislative mechanisms for reimbursement of low vision services are presently at a minimum, the concept of low vision services and their benefit to the visually impaired person is increasing. Visually impaired consumers are becoming more aware of low vision services, of their own needs, and of the fact that they have usable vision. As the need increases for these services, legislators will be held accountable by their supporters for developing appropriate legislation. However, the appropriate legislative mechanisms will not occur by themselves. It is doubtful that a useful legislative program will develop through the efforts of a single agency or organization. There is a need for the organizations and agencies delivering rehabilitative care to the visually impaired to form a coalition with consumer groups. This will provide uniformity and agreement within the field, adding to the national political clout that is required to force legislators to take a serious look at these needs.

More and more private insurance companies are offering health packages that cover low vision services. The reimbursement is usually covered through the major medical rider. It may be possible that when our legislators finally consider developing a national program, incentive mechanisms will be developed for private insurance companies to include low vision services. This would reduce the burden on existing legislative programs with limited budgets such as Medicare. By developing private insurance incentives to include low vision care, there would also be peripheral advantages, such as developing greater employer and consumer interest in these programs, which would in turn cause a greater demand for more comprehensive insurance programs in a competitive environment.

The need to develop greater consumer awareness about low vision care cannot be overemphasized. Some stereotypes and misconceptions about vision impairment within the general optometric and ophthalmological communities still persist. The educated consumer must play a major part in causing the actual changes in low vision referrals and service delivery to occur by setting no geographic limits in their search for visual rehabilitation and becoming vocal about their needs within their communities. As a result, more professionals will begin to pay attention to the low vision rehabilitation needs of their patients.

Agencies for the blind and visually impaired are also becoming more aware of the concept of low vision services. Some have developed low vision clinics within their agencies. The majority refer visually impaired individuals to private practitioners specializing in low vision and low vision clinics.

It has been interesting to observe the redirection and growth of many professions historically involved in the field of blindness. As low vision services have become a recognized means of rehabilitation, many of the professions have adapted to the concept of "vision" instead of the strictly limited "blindness" concept, which restricted the ability to offer a rehabilitation service that more completely met the needs of their clients. As concepts were reoriented to include the visually impaired individual's use of his remaining vision, the depth to which the profession could delve in new areas of research and rehabilitation became unlimited. In many ways the concept of low vision services and maximizing use of residual vision has been a breakthrough not only for the visually impaired but also for those professions serving them. The author believes that within the next 20 years, this breakthrough will cause new horizons to be set within individual professions as they each become more comfortable with concepts of vision as opposed to blindness. This will also cause an increased demand for more professionals in these fields, thus ending the past decade's limited manpower growth.

As the demand increases for services, and after a legislative mechanism is in place, industry will develop new and improved aids. This is beginning to occur with the transfer of high technology to companies interested in low vision rehabilitation. Most recent advancements have been in electronic devices. Many of these devices are cumbersome, first-generation products. It is expected that their bulkiness will be overcome as technology is refined. Also, the technology of electro-optics (the combination of electronics and refined optics) for the purpose of image referral remains an untapped area for visual rehabilitation. Most of the research and development is involved in the development of microscopes and telescopes for use in surgery. As this technology becomes refined and simplified, it is quite possible that a new generation of aids will be developed for visually impaired individuals.

While there is much work to be done to develop both the concept of low vision services and the means to deliver appropriate interdisciplinary services to meet the needs of visually impaired persons, the future is far from bleak. The field of low vision will expand for individual professions and will be the impetus for cooperation between professions. It is critical, however, that those involved in developing new directions be responsible for developing directions that are complementary to, rather than encroaching upon, the services offered by other professions.

CHAPTER IX

ENHANCING VISION AND MOTOR SKILLS IN THE LEARNING ENVIRONMENT

Learning is adaptation. "Adaptation is described as an organized process of modification in which an individual assimilates everything that is happening, accommodates to these experiences and associates, differentiates and integrates the new experience with those previously acquired" (Gilfoyle et al, 1981).

In normal development a child learns early to prepare to respond. He begins to organize random movements and reflexes into postural strategies to prepare his body for subsequent movement. In other words, the child learns to support purposeful activity with postural readiness. He also learns to anticipate new information and feedback from his response. He participates in a new experience; he learns. As he develops, he continues to modify and integrate postural strategies and purposeful activity into more complex, learned behaviors. To illustrate this concept, consider the three-month-old infant who sights a toy (sensory input). In response to seeing, the child swipes at the toy (motor output) and moves it into closer range. The child's efforts are rewarded as he can now more closely examine the toy, better feel its properties, and realize that he has effectively acted upon his environment. Because the child has associated, or learned, that purposeful movement brings accomplishment and success, he is reinforced and encouraged to repeat the activity. More complex and differentiated behaviors emerge. Guided by vision, his swipe is refined into direct reach, and direct reach later combines with controlled grasp and manipulation to allow for retrieval and control of objects.

Throughout development the motor system depends on a reliable sensory system to feed it. The visual system both enhances and is the catalyst for motor development, until the motor system overrides and becomes the catalyst for visual development. The motor system gives movement responses that become new sensory experiences. Finally, the visual and motor systems are intertwined in the growth and maturation of the individual. They continually augment one another to direct later development. These experiences provide the developing system with feedback which is synthesized and associated with similar experiences.

When children are unable, due to disability, to receive information (sensory dysfunction) or to react (motor dysfunction), extrinsic structuring becomes necessary. Educators are faced with the task of structuring the environment to allow for maximum functioning and efficient learning to occur. Postural preparation, or positioning, is basic to environmental structuring, allowing the receiving-reacting process to occur. The utilization of positioning becomes an initial and essential part of the structuring process. The goal of positioning is to facilitate efficient performance of the sensory-motor system, capturing and directing energy into meaningful activity, to allow maximum function with minimal pathology. Simply put, stress on the system is reduced, thereby allowing for optimal performance. It is against this background that education should take place.

Assessment is the initial step in the rehabilitation process. The assessment will compile information that should describe the developmental status of the total child. Problems in learning, as they relate to disability and impairment, must be identified. Later, assessment results are utilized to formulate the plan of remediation.

An appropriate protocol for assessment employs the concept of environmental structuring by:

1. establishing postural (motor), attitudinal and emotional readiness;

2. selecting relevant tasks and materials to allow for motivation and success;

3.   providing familiar, non-threatening physical space free of distractions and disturbances.

Throughout the assessment it is paramount that the child be allowed freedom of expression to demonstrate his preferred methods and styles of learning. The identification of problems and strengths should always be qualified by the way the child approaches and executes learning tasks. Thus, assessment results become descriptive and provide the educator with more meaningful information. The "style of learning," as displayed by the child during assessment, becomes an essential element in planning the educational program. Assessment must be viewed as an ongoing process, wherein specific samples of behavior are gathered over a period of time, providing a comprehensive picture of strengths and weaknesses. It is important to apply these elements of general assessment to each specific area of concern-- in this case, sight and vision.

The traditional vision assessment provides information on the physical impairment, the overall medical status of the eye, as well as the visual acuities and the visual field as measured against a norm. This information provides baseline data and gains educational significance only when incorporated as a component of the functional vision assessment. In the functional vision assessment, we view the eye specialists' reports at a point of "stability." The specialists make all of the changes possible medically and optically (in the traditional sense) so that sight is stabilized and the impairment minimized. The disability is determined by the extent to which the stabilized impairment interferes with function. It is then possible to have a particular level of impairment result in varying levels of disability. For example, two children with the same diagnosis and accurately measured 20/200 acuities can function at vastly different levels of performance. One child adapts well and succeeds, while the other experiences difficulty and frequent failure. For one child, the impairment is far more disabling than for the other in that it more seriously interferes with his function. As professionals, we realize that modifications can be made in the classroom environment, the assigned activities, and the learning materials which will enhance or disturb the child's performance. In accomplishing our goal of maximizing function, we are actually changing the level of disability.

Knowing that change can occur, we provide a rationale for intervention. By intervening upon the developing systems, we facilitate their capacity to modify or compensate for impairment. This causes further adaptations to be made and additional learned behaviors can then emerge. Intervention should provide experiences for meaningful sensory reception and opportunities for functional motor response. This allows for more normalized sensory feedback, and system maturation, or learning, results.

To further insure that such intervention is meaningful, both the learning task and the learning environment should approximate that of actual function. "Educators have systematically, although inadvertently, impaired many handicapped and non-handicapped students from acquiring the skills, values, and attitudes necessary to function in heterogeneous and complex environments" (Brown, Nietupski & Hamre-Nietupski, 1976). Since the time needed to acquire skills is expanded and the ability to generalize skills is more limited, following a functional curriculum model is vital when programming for severely handicapped students. For less severely handicapped students, the functional curriculum increases relevant to learning opportunities.

To implement a functional approach, the professional team must project into the child's future using developmental guidelines. The goals and objectives should be under close scrutiny by all team members. As a skill is acquired, new variables are introduced. These familiar tasks with new variables encourage and allow the child to make comparisons and generalize the skill to future situations.

Programming is no longer limited to a traditional classroom base but can and should include consideration of the child's school, home and community environments. The curriculum must be expanded to include vocational leisure and independent life skills. This expanded view of classroom and curriculum increases opportunities for enhancing the overall development of the child and greatly impacts the quality of his life.

This approach to education necessitates a critical look at the materials, equipment and media used in the classroom. An object itself is used rather than a commercial product that appears real. Consider the teacher working with naming food items such as fruit. Rather than provide pictures or plastic models, she demonstrates with fresh fruit. The child can then experience the tactile, olfactory and visual attributes of each piece of fruit. Materials used in the classroom should be carefully chosen in the same way that the learning environment and teaching methods are selected. Relevant, functional and multiple-use items should be chosen to assure transfer of the skills learned.

An additional benefit of this approach comes as a result of having the teaching and learning occur in the functional environment. Actual problems are addressed as they arise, and the effectiveness of the specialized staff is maximized. Performing tasks in the functional environment provides the opportunity for independent, individualized, or small group learning. Specialized education is no longer limited to one-to-one intervention. This flexibility relies upon the structuring of the intervention environment, allowing for optimal performance on the part of the professionals as well as the students.

When planning for the remediation of visual disabilities, we view visual functioning as a learned behavior. While vision is present at birth, the infant does not see and perceive as the adult does (Corbin 1980). Throughout the normal developmental sequence, the child is given many opportunities to expand and refine visual skills and to integrate the visual system with the other systems of his being. Impairment of any system on any level interferes with the child's natural maturation. Since visual functioning is a learned behavior, visual skills can be taught. Considering that over 70 percent of the input we receive and process comes through the visual channel (Padula & Spungin 1982), this is an overwhelming responsibility. However, when children with poor skills in visual functioning are given carefully structured opportunities to experience and integrate sensory input, marked improvement is demonstrated. Activities to increase visual skills are developed in response to the functional visual assessment against the backdrop of the child's abilities and needs, with overall function as the ultimate goal. One of the major tasks of the professional who interacts with visually impaired children is that of coordinating resource personnel into a unit that works to meet the comprehensive needs of the child. This might best be accomplished by following a transdisciplinary model of service delivery. Assessments can be carried out by individual specialists, but direct service is provided by one or two persons. Other team members provide supportive consultation. Emphasis is on sharing information, and the general knowledge base for all team members is increased. Consultants can train the primary care providers in the necessary skills to carry out team programming goals (Albano, et al. 1981).

Because of the close tie between vision and motor skills, and because intervention in one area will influence the other, the educator will find it necessary to carefully orchestrate services between vision and motor specialists. For example, the classroom teacher, serving as the "primary" educator for a multiple- impaired child, may find that input from the vision specialist and the physical/occupational therapist is needed for activities when the child is in a sitting position. The vision specialist determines how the student best functions with sight and vision; that is, she identifies his optimal visual learning style. The vision specialist then selects specific materials and offers suggestions for their presentation and incorporation in programming, thereby increasing opportunities for the efficient use of vision. The physical and occupational therapists assess the child's "motor picture" and determine how posture and mobility can be enhanced to improve overall function. The occupational therapist designs appropriate facilitation of upper body function to enable accurate reach and grasp. The physical therapist arranges for proper positioning to insure symmetry, stability and, ultimately, head control. The classroom teacher then utilizes the input from all three professionals in planning for the myriad tasks she will teach requiring activity at a desk or table. Thus, functioning can be enhanced with extrinsic postural correction or intrinsic postural control, coupled with visual efficiency. Together, vision and motor specialists provide teachers with valuable information that assists them in structuring the learning environment for maximum function. Because improved function is achieved, learning experiences are increased and overall development is enhanced.

Realizing the importance of integrating the visual and motor systems to achieve optimal function, it becomes obvious that therapists and teachers of the visually impaired must be well versed in both of these areas to successfully meet student needs. Programs preparing these professionals generally provide sufficient background in vision or motor skills, leaving the specialist unprepared to deal with the critical alternate issues.

There are numerous courses available that relate to sensory-motor areas, including those offered through orientation and mobility certification, physical education departments, nursing and science programs. While such courses can provide excellent information, they do not quite meet the overall need in that they are too specific to other concerns and leave the specialist responsible to synthesize and appropriately apply the information on a day-to-day basis.

In actuality, the need is for teacher-therapists, yet it is often not practical or desirable to have a specialist cross over entirely into an alternate profession. All of the members of the transdisciplinary team must have knowledge and understanding of the generic processes of vision and movement as they apply to all skill domains (Campbell 1982). Teachers and therapists alike would do well to participate in training programs that are neurodevelopmental in nature, while emphasizing the team approach to insure the students' successful performance in functional activities.

As noted earlier, the results of the assessment provide the educational team with the information necessary to formulate the plan of intervention. When planning remediation or intervention, there are several additional factors to consider. Within a motor framework, the child is viewed as a closed energy system, one in which the total amount of usable energy is divided throughout the various systems that the child must use to accomplish a task. At any one time, if we can conserve some of the energy expenditure from one system and redirect it to another system, we can further enable a challenged system to function. For example, the four-month-old child expends energy to achieve and sustain the prone position. The demand to perform a new task in this position, such as fixating on specific objects, creates an energy deficit. The educator intervenes by alleviating stress on one system by placing the child in a semi-supine position. This change in posture allows for the redirection of energy toward the fixation task.

Another consideration in planning intervention is establishing a postural set, or positioning the child in a state of readiness to perform. Optimal preparation of the body for sensory reception allows for more efficient movement responses. Thus, the utilization of positioning, or securing the child's position in space, maximizes the potential for learning.

While positioning can provide the additional support needed to improve posture and performance, it will not provide the motivation. For example, proper positioning will make it easier (or possible) for the child to lift his head but will not give him a reason to do so (Campbell 1984). The educator's role is not limited to identifying problem areas and designing solutions, but must also include planning for the child's active participation in the remediation process.

Motivation is related in part to the previous experiences with which the child approaches an activity. This mind set includes the store of knowledge that the child has accumulated over time and the expectations he has of the task and its outcome. Past experiences can be motor, sensory, cognitive, and/or emotional in nature and can be drawn upon to enrich the learning experience.

The issue of motivation also applies to staff needs. The team must continually generate new ideas for improving service delivery and insuring continuity of treatment from one team member to the next.

Programming that moves beyond the formal report stage to incorporate the personal aspect, while insuring that all team members are aware of programming decisions, can serve to meet current needs while stimulating future team input and emphasizing the student as a participant (see Figure 3).

Finally, it is important to realize that, simultaneous to the development of visual functioning, the child, as a complex, multisystem entity, is developing, maturing, learning and improving. The systems play off one another--none occurs in isolation. Activities directed toward incorporating more than a single system enhance not only the systems involved in the activity, but also the child's ability to integrate sensory information. The goal is not to achieve a dominance of one sensory modality over another, but rather to achieve a balance between the systems. When balance is achieved, the child is better able to discriminate and integrate sensory input.

One can readily identify the interdependence between the sensory and motor systems. Because sight, and ultimately vision, is the dominating sense drawing the child into and guiding him through his environment, the educator serving children with visual disabilities must address the visual and motor systems simultaneously. In addition, other areas of development (cognitive, language, social and emotional) cannot be overlooked in planning educational programs intended to address the needs of the child as a whole. Skilled professionals, teachers and therapists increase knowledge and improve service via cooperation with fellow team members in a transdisciplinary approach to education. Assessment and remediation occur in an environment structured to emphasize function which, when achieved, will serve to significantly decrease, if not dissolve, the disabling nature of the child's impairment.

Figure 3.
Presentation of a Classroom Program

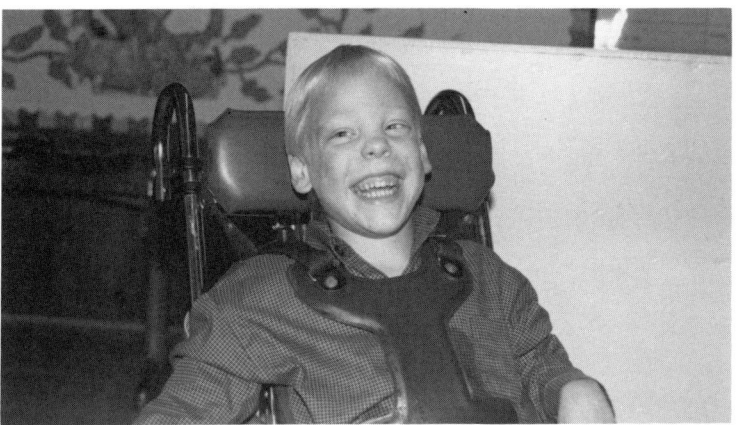

Hi! My name is Quentin W..

I can see light and bright, shiny things that move. I might be able to see shadows, if they are simple and clear. I can move my eyes all around, but sometimes it is difficult for me to control where my eyes decide to look. I can use both of my eyes, but have trouble seeing clearly. I like it when the things I'm looking at move or make noise.

My position is very important to how well I can work with my eyes, arms and hands. I do best in my prone stander. It is the easiest place for me to work. With the tray on, you can put things in front of me so that I can look at them. I like to look at and reach for things hanging on my mobile, although sometimes I'll need your help for reaching out.

There are lots of things I need to work on, but it is very important that I improve my head control. If I can learn to look more often and more correctly, it might help me to improve faster. It is easiest for me to work on good head control when I'm in my new Rifton chair or my special wheelchair.

I am also working with a joy-stick switch. I use my right hand to activate it. Sometimes I use the switch when I'm sitting in my wheelchair. Then it is important that the wheelchair be as straight up as possible, with the tray as low as possible, so that I can reach out to work the switch.

Best Place to Put Things:

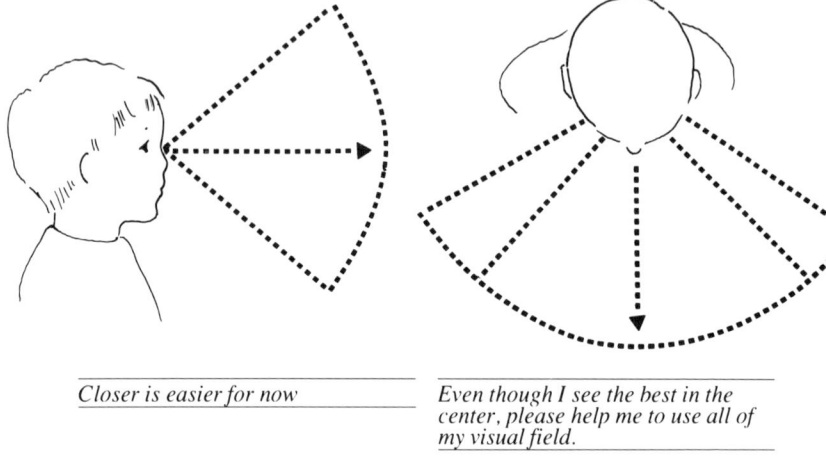

Closer is easier for now

Even though I see the best in the center, please help me to use all of my visual field.

Ideas:
- Give me lots of BIG, SHINY, NOISY, MOVING things to look at.
- Pair my "vision toys" with sound or touch--or both.
- Tell me what we are doing.
- Help me to move my head in the right direction.
- Try backlighting shapes for me to see.
- Show me things close up, then slowly move them to see if I can follow with my eyes.
- Show me things, then help me to move my hands to touch and move the things I look at.

Besides me, the other members of my team are Laurel, Gwen and Kathleen. If you have any questions, just ask one of us for help!

CHAPTER X

LOW VISION AND EDUCATION FOR THE SCHOOL-AGE CHILD

Rehabilitation for the visually impaired person has been greatly enhanced since the development of the low vision examination 30 to 40 years ago. Prior to that development, simple magnifiers were used in a trial and error approach with little or no scientific methodology. The use of magnifiers was not considered part of rehabilitation, and it was left primarily up to the visually impaired person to find an appropriate magnifier. In many cases, it was not until adulthood that an individual even used magnifiers.

Long ago, the term "blind" for the visually impaired child was more than just a classification. It de-emphasized the importance of vision. Educational and rehabilitation programs emphasized development of tactual and auditory skills to compensate for the supposed lack of vision. The school age child with a vision impairment was isolated from children who didn't have physical impairments. "Sight-saving" classrooms and schools for the blind were established. Braille was taught and auditory training given because it was thought that further use of vision would cause its eventual loss. Children were actually discouraged from using their vision.

This brief historical review should not be thought of as criticism of the methods that were used. The purpose of these introductory paragraphs is to set a stage so that the reader can understand why our current philosophies and understandings have developed and be able to recognize the importance of the low vision services for the visually impaired child.

When it was recognized that optical aids could actually be beneficial to habilitating the use of residual vision, methodology was developed to equate the magnification needs of the patient with acuity measurements and visual field. The low vision examination during these early years utilized a concept of vision that did not always relate to function. The static measurements of acuity and field are related more to the optical considerations than they are to the functional abilities and/or potentials of the person.

Initially, though, as many individuals became visually rehabilitated, the philosophy for saving sight began to change, and the visual abilities of the patient were emphasized. Programs to improve the visual efficiency of the child were developed. Clinical and experimental research proved that not only could visual functioning be improved, but that vision would not deteriorate further (Barraga 1969).

Although the concept of a low vision examination gained recognition as an attempt to improve visual functioning of the school-age child, success was limited. Criteria were developed for appropriate referrals that related to age and acuity measurements. It was not until it was understood that there was more to visual functioning than an acuity or field measurement, that the concept of low vision and the provision of services began to change. Clinicians found that, given similar pathological conditions, acuities and visual field, some individuals functioned as if there were almost no impairment, while others were almost totally visually debilitated.

An understanding of the dynamic qualities of vision from observation and clinical and experimental research led the clinician away from the optical model of low vision to a concept that is more rehabilitative and need-oriented. This does not mean simply asking the patient about what his needs are, but rather attempting to understand visual function by observing behavior. Behavior represents the way the individual utilizes the visual process to lead motor function.

Optical aids alone do not improve visual function. Acuity may improve but is not an indication of improved function. The optical aid is a tool. If the process of vision can utilize this tool effectively, function can be improved.

The low vision examination has evolved to include new methodology that is adaptive to the needs of the visually impaired child. In addition, new modes of electro-diagnostic testing enable the clinician to analyze and detect pathology to new depths. Assessment of visual function in the habitual environment is also recognized as an integral part of the low vision analysis. Information about visual functioning in the home, classroom, and/or environment enables the clinician to establish more meaning to the acuity and field measurements in the office setting. In order to accomplish this, educators and rehabilitation professionals can perform functional assessments in the field and relay this information to the clinician.

The information gathered can greatly assist the clinician in determining the most appropriate prescriptive optical aids for the child. Further, training programs for learning to use the aids and improving visual function can be moved from the office setting to the habitual environment of the child. This way, a follow-through is developed that enables the clinician to develop an effective means of low vision habilitation for the child. The follow-through by the educator and/or rehabilitation professional also enables the child to be referred back for further clinical assessment and prescriptive devices should some aspect of behavioral function change.

The present concept of low vision includes a multidisciplinary philosophy which recognizes that the needs of the visually impaired child cannot be met by one professional alone. However, it is best if the clinician remains the hub of this service.

The functional abilities of the child should be assessed using varied methods and settings in order to determine the child's critical needs. By utilizing a multidisciplinary approach, a cross perspective of those needs can be established which give the clinician greater insight into the most effective means of prescribing and designing appropriate training programs for the child. This concept has caused low vision to evolve from solely an examination and prescription of optical aids to a model of service that includes educators and rehabilitation professionals. In the low vision service model, functional assessment, clinical assessment, prescription, adaptive training, referral and follow-up are the keys to success. While the low vision clinical examination remains the integral part of this service model, the clinician must understand that success will be determined by improved performance and not increased acuity. Further, the involvement of the educator and rehabilitation professional will increase the potential for success of visual habilitation.

The de-emphasis on acuity relating to improved function has already been made but must be clarified further. Acuity and field measurements still represent an important quantitative measurement taken by the clinician of the visually impaired child. Certainly, refractive corrections and predicted magnification systems should and will continue to be made in the clinical assessment. However, a dynamic, qualitative understanding of the visual process of the child must be given greater attention. The acuity measurement is really a function of the visual process. The ability to visually control and manipulate an aspect of the field yields the acuity measurement.

Vision and its process can affect the child's overall development. Vision is a dynamic, interactive process of motor and sensory function mediated by the eyes for the purpose of manipulating and controlling the external environment and thought. Therefore, the clinician must attempt to analyze how the child utilizes his vision in a manner that relates to habitual environmental settings, i.e., the classroom. The visual skills used in the classroom, such as near-far fixations, saccadic fixations, spatial relationships, eye-hand coordination, balance and motor coordination, must be analyzed by the clinician. These visual functions should be evaluated as part of the low vision examination so that the clinician can determine where the visual interferences occur and impact these interferences by developing appropriate habilitative programming.

For example, a 10-year-old visually impaired boy with 20/80 acuity, central serous retinopathy, and no peripheral field loss was referred for a low vision examination by an educator. The reason for referral was the need to improve the child's ability to see the chalkboard for the purpose of copying assignments and taking notes. The functional assessment performed by the educator noted that the child often became disoriented in the classroom. The prescription of a telescope was first considered. In this case a testing situation was developed using large printed letters cut into two vertical strips and mounted on a wall approximately three feet apart. The child was positioned approximately four feet from the charts and asked to read a letter from each strip, thereby showing saccadic fixations. Similar testing was designed for near-far fixation ability using a large block of letters mounted on a wall 10 feet from the child and a block of printed letters on a card that the child held. The child was asked to read one letter from each chart alternately.

The tests revealed that the child frequently lost his place and quickly became frustrated with the tasks. While acuity measurements with a 4.0x hand-held telescope were improved from 20/20 to 20/40+, the child became very disoriented. Even without the telescope, the child demonstrated difficulty using his vision to orient himself in his environment and using peripheral visual cues to orient central visual functions. The functional assessment by the educator hinted at this, and the clinical assessment further revealed this interference which extended beyond acuity loss.

To prescribe a telescope that would magnify and reduce the visual field would further limit the ability of the child to utilize peripheral visual cues. Therefore, it was decided that the educational program should compensate for these difficulties initially. Adaptive habilitative programs would then be developed to minimize the visual interferences and improve the child's visual functioning to a level at which a telescope could be prescribed.

It was recommended that copying activities be limited to copying from a paper on the child's desk rather than from the chalkboard. Seating in the classroom was changed so that the child was positioned in the front row. In addition, a training program began that included localizing the sound of a bell by pointing toward the bell with eyes closed, then opening the eyes to correct and reinforce.

The pointing served to give kinesthetic reinforcement to establish visual and auditory direction. The purpose of the activity was to develop the integrative process of vision.

As progress was made, activities were developed that included near-far fixations and saccadic fixations at varying distances. With these activities, the child used a flashlight to point to the object or letter he was looking at, again to develop kinesthetic reinforcement. When progress was noted, a cardboard tube was introduced that limited peripheral vision. At first, a large tube offering a minimal field limitation was used, and then the field was reduced using smaller-diameter tubes as progress was made.

These activities were performed by the teacher of the visually impaired child several times a week, and monthly check-ups on progress were made by the clinician. Within four months, a wide-angle telescope was introduced, and training was started in the office and continued by the educator. Within six months the child's skills were improved to the extent that the original 4.0x hand-held telescope was prescribed for use in the classroom.

Early Low Vision Intervention

The clinician must consider developmental aspects when performing a low vision examination since delays in development may interfere with success. Through appropriate low vision habilitation programming, the practitioner may actually be able to influence the child's development.

The development of the child is a function of three variables: physical abilities, psychological disposition and environmental influences. Vision is not isolated in one variable but actually is part of all three. It certainly has a physical nature and it includes perceptual aspects, but it is also influenced by the environment.

If a child with a visual impairment has adequate or above-average intellectual and perceptual abilities and is placed in a stimulating environment, he may be able to compensate for the physical/visual deficit to maintain development.

Conversely, if the child cannot compensate for his physical deficit, a delay in development may occur. Even though a child may be chronologically seven years old, his developmental age may only be four or five years. In this case, the practitioner should expect the behavior and functional abilities of a younger child. The clinical implications are that the practitioner may need to consider establishing both short- and long-range objectives from the low vision examination. Simple magnifiers may be effective initially to improve general functioning at near ranges. Special training programs may be necessary, however, to improve the visual skills in order to utilize more sophisticated devices such as spectacle-mounted microscope prescriptions and/or hand-held telescopes.

When the practitioner encounters a child whot may be developmentally delayed, several symptoms may be apparent when discussing the history with the educator and/or parent. The child may be a behavioral problem in school, being unable to stay seated for a long period or exhibiting frequent loss of attention and concentration. Sometimes the parent and/or educator may misperceive these symptoms and state that the child is lazy or doesn't work up to potential.

The practitioner should not assume that the lack of ability to see clearly is the reason the child is not functioning up to expectations. In this case the parent and/or educator may think that the prescribed optical aid will solve the problem, when in fact the child's lack of developmental-perceptual abilities may interfere with the use of the aid. Failure to use the aid properly and/or no change in the child's behavior in the classroom may cause the educator and parent to view the low vision examination as a failure.

The practitioner must attempt to differentiate the developmental difficulties from those difficulties caused by acuity interruption. To do this, the history should include a discussion of developmental milestones such as the age the child crawled, walked, and spoke in phrases and sentences. Perceptual-motor testing of balance and motor integration should give the practitioner a general idea of whether the child is behind in expected abilities related to chronological norms. In addition, some developmental tests such as the Gesell Copy Forms Test, Incomplete Man Test, or the Beary Test may be given. Although these tests may need to be adapted somewhat by darkening lines, etc., to meet the visual abilities of the child, the general developmental age level scored on these tests may be helpful in understanding the child's behaviors and abilities.

When a child has developmental interferences, the practitioner should spend time explaining the implications to both the parents and the educator. Extra school work assignments or homework will not serve the child's best interests. What is needed is habilitative programming designed to improve the child's skills and thereby affect his functioning and development.

A complete review of all aspects of designing an appropriate habilitative program cannot be developed within the confines of this chapter. The practitioner should, however, understand that the child's development is greatly influenced by the visual process. Therefore, the key to affecting development lies in improving the visual skills in areas of fixation, pursuit tracking, saccadic fixations, and perceptual-motor abilities. Since the developmental process involves the use of vision to lead motor functions and match information between vision and other senses, habilitative programs must include training the child to utilize the visual process to match information between sensory and motor systems.

The results of this type of habilitative programming may not be immediate but may take months of consistent training. It is most effective for the practitioner to be directly involved in leading the training and changing programming when necessary. The parent and the educator can and should be involved in carrying out procedures on a daily basis. Prescription of optical aids may need to be limited to the child's abilities until visual skill levels have been improved. At that time more sophisticated devices may be given.

The First Low Vision Examination
A question often asked by educators and parents is how old the child should be to refer for a low vision examination. When taking

into consideration the developmental nature of the visual process, the answer to this question varies. The practitioner in low vision should be consulted as soon as possible after the visual impairment is diagnosed because he may be able to prescribe spectacles, contact lenses, bifocals, and even optical aids that will affect the overall development. Also, long-range planning can be started concerning the child's future needs. For example, if it is anticipated that a three-year-old child will require spotting telescopes for classroom use in the future, the preschool educator of the visually handicapped may be trained in spotting techniques, and additional habilitative programming may be developed. It is also imperative that medical and/or surgical intervention be considered as soon as possible if it will improve the visual state of the child.

In discussing the needs of the visually impaired child with groups of educators and/or parents, the optometrist must stress the importance of early referral for low vision services. Often a child is not referred until he is eight years of age or older. Too many years may have passed in the child's life before an effective visual program, including refractive corrections and low vision devices, can be developed.

One young man was referred at the age of 16 for his first low vision examination. He had spastic cerebral palsy and was confined to a wheelchair. When he was three years old he was classified as legally blind because acuity testing with best correction did not yield results better than 20/200. Since that time, no visual examinations had been performed. Upon examining this young man, 4 diopters of myopia was objectively determined. The subjective refraction improved his acuity from 20/200 to 20/50, demonstrating that he was not legally blind. Educators and parents should recognize that the low vision examination can, even through only the refraction, greatly improve the child's visual abilities.

This approach may enable the low vision practitioner to describe aids to very young children. If aids are prescribed for the preschool child, acceptance is greater. Essentially, the child will grow up with the aids as part of his life. Also, peer pressure in preschool is less than at elementary school levels. By the time the child reaches elementary school, he will have learned to cope with peer pressure situations that will undoubtedly arise.

How the young child will adapt to situations is demonstrated by one who had been using aids since he was three years old. He obviously felt that his aids were important. On his first day in the first grade, he took out a 2.5x hand-held spotting telescope to see what his teacher looked like. He told several surprised children who approached him just how things would be when he said, "The first one who makes fun of my telescope, I'm gonna deck." While not all children would deal with the situation as "tactfully" as he did, most children who have used optical aids since preschool will continue to use them throughout their school years and beyond. An older child just receiving aids, however, may not be able to effectively deal with peer influences.

The teacher of the visually impaired can be very effective in dealing with problems that arise in school over the use of optical aids. Initially, the teacher may go directly into the classroom and give a presentation to the other children about what a vision impairment is and what optical aids are for. The children may even be permitted to try the aids to develop their understanding.

Prescription glasses and aids for the preschool child should not be based solely on improvement in acuity. Often, if the practitioner detects a moderate or even a low amount of myopia, hyperopia, or astigmatism, no prescription will be given if a significant improvement in acuity is not demonstrated. If the practitioner were to evaluate perceptual-motor skills and touch- point ability (ability to reach and localize an object accurately), the effects of the lenses might be more readily observed.

Measuring Success

The utilization of optical aids in the practitioner's office should not be considered a success in habilitating the patient. There are too many factors in the classroom and/or home environment that can interfere. The service can only be considered successful after the child has demonstrated improved function and performance in the habitual setting. This can be determined only after a follow-up examination and/or communication with the educator and parent.

The relative nature of success is demonstrated by one 10-year-old girl who had undifferentiated maculas in both eyes, a moderate amount of hyperopia (OU), and nystagmus. She was referred for a low vision examination to determine whether optical aids would be effective in improving her ability to read and see the chalkboard. The result of the examination determined that her acuity at near improved from 20/120 to 20/30 with a 4x stand magnifier. A hand magnifier was prescribed to enable her visual flexibility at intermediate ranges to be used particularly for her science course. Bifocal lenses were prescribed due to her distance and near vision improvement. A hand-held telescope improved her distance vision from 10/80 to 10/30, and she demonstrated proficient use of all three aids after being trained for 30 minutes in the office.

The novelty of the aids soon became worn, and her teacher reported that the girl would not use them or the glasses because several children made fun of her. The teacher of the visually impaired girl attempted to remedy the situation by talking with the other children about vision impairment. Although the ridicule stopped, the girl still refused to use the aids.

Through follow-up visits with the low vision practitioner and communication among the educator, optometrist, parent, and social worker, progress began by having the girl use the aids only at home. Several of her friends began to ask her why she wasn't using her glasses, and for short periods she began to wear them in school. After one year of continued low vision service, the girl began to use the aids in school. Her grades improved and this appeared to reinforce her use of the aids. For this child the initial demonstration that she could use the aids was a false sense of success. The true measurement of success was only achieved after a year of follow-through low vision service by additional professionals.

Success for another child was measured in a different way. A three-year-old boy was referred for a low vision evaluation. He had spastic cerebral palsy, was previously diagnosed as cortically blind, and speech was not evident. His previous doctor told the mother that her child could see somewhat, but that there was nothing that could help him.

Upon performing the evaluation, it was determined that the child was able to fixate on a puppet for two to three seconds at approximately a one-foot range. Tracking movements were not elicited, and horizontal saccadic fixations were observed between two lights approximately five inches apart. Reaching for an object was found to be inconsistent and inaccurate. Acuity testing was unreliable. Distance retinoscopy revealed 2 diopters of hyperopia in both eyes and near (Bell) retinoscopy found with motion (no accommodative response) at near ranges. When the hyperopia correction was introduced, intermittent against motion reflexes were monitored when he fixated at a 10- inch range. With these lenses, fixation increased to eight to nine seconds and brief tracking movements were made.

Lenses were prescribed for the purpose of investigating their effects on the child's performance. They were to be worn for one- or two-hour periods. Several activities were developed for the child to be performed by the mother. These activities included tracking an object that was placed in his hand while his mother moved his hand passively at first and then attempted to stimulate his active movement. Also, activities were developed to encourage reach and touch. A functional means of testing acuity was developed by the optometrist and carried out daily by the parent.

After three months the parent returned with the child and reported that behavioral changes had been noted in the child's posture and in his awareness. His mother stated that after the first week she noticed that he did not slump in his chair when wearing the lenses for the recommended periods of time. The follow-up evaluation revealed that his fixation period with the glasses had improved to up to thirty seconds, and that he was able to track horizontally and in a circle. Near (Bell) retinoscopy found against motion reflex sustained during fixation at 10 inches. His reach and object localization improved considerably at an eight-inch range, and he also seemed to fixate on objects around the room. Also, behavioral observations of visual fixation and attention at home enabled the optometrist to equate an acuity of approximately 20/100 (OU).

For this young boy success was not based solely on the quantitative measurements of retinoscopy, but was measured on a qualitative assessment of the child's performance over a period of time. It is difficult for many practitioners to provide qualitative assessments of vision since educational programs for optometric training emphasize quantitative testing. For many visually impaired children, however, quantitative measurements offer little advantage. In this case the behavioral changes from the prescriptive lenses represented progress that the parent had not previously seen. This progress, although it may have been slight in comparison to another child, represented major advancements in his use of vision.

The practitioner should approach the evaluation of low functioning children such as this young boy in an investigative, observational manner that attempts to analyze how the child uses his vision. A complete analysis of the use of vision, whether there are peripheral or central scotomas, what the visual acuity is, etc., cannot be completed during the first visit and actually may take months or even years of repeated assessment. It is often beneficial to design functional testing activities for acuity and visual field to be performed daily at home by the parent so that an averaging of behavioral responses can be made and compared with the child's next visit to the practitioner's office.

The Parent

The home environment is a valuable component in forming a comprehensive view of the needs of the visually impaired child. The parents' role in this aspect of the low vision evaluation is important. How a parent views his child's impairment and what he understands of it reflect his attitude and give insight as to how the family is coping with it at home.

The parent must have a good understanding of the purpose of the low vision evaluation. Many parents will experience this concept for the first time with their child. The clinician may meet with some skepticism, or an unrealistic expectation, for example, that the child will "regain" sight. It should not be taken for granted that the parent has a good background of the pathology of his child's visual impairment. Although a parent may have a complete and positive understanding of his child's impairment, there are those who for years have been told that nothing more could be done. Therefore, they have been asked to understand and accept the child's "blindness," de-emphasizing residual vision and any hope for rehabilitation.

A parent cannot be expected to have an objective view of his child's visual impairment. Some are able to perceive a relationship between the impairment and the child's abilities and limitations. Others, perhaps being overprotective, tend to misperceive the relationship of the pathology to function and project limitations upon the child based on their inaccurate notion of the impairment. Still others may underemphasize the impairment, pretending it does not exist, thus presenting a possible barrier to accepting that rehabilitation is needed. In discussing parental views, one can recognize the effort that must be made to form positive, cohesive relationships between clinician and parent, a task which takes time.

The practitioner must be aware that there are circumstances in parent/child relationships that will in fact interfere with the low vision examination process. The parent may view his visually impaired child as lacking in abilities or being very fragile, resulting in overprotectiveness. The child who has overly cautious parents may have had very limited opportunity to explore and experience his environment. This in turn may affect development and the child's self-image. The child may feel inadequate as a result of not being given the chance to succeed, or even fail at a particular task. These kinds of undertones may cause negative results to occur in the low vision examination. And despite the practitioner's efforts, the optical aid(s) alone may not be the solution to the problem.

The practitioner must be sensitive to situations where the parent may expect too much of the low vision examination. Failure to change behavior may be interpreted by the parent as failure of the examination.

The practitioner may be alerted to an overprotective parent during history taking. The parent and child should be asked about the child's self-help abilities, such as his personal hygiene skills, grooming and dressing skills, and assisting around the house (i.e., cleaning, cooking, setting the table). The overprotective parent will usually respond that the child is unable to perform these tasks independently, when in fact the child has been given very little opportunity to develop these skills. The interview might also reveal a situation where the parent consistently answers for the child. This indicates that the parent is allowing the child little exposure to varied situations. The practitioner, in discussing parent/child relationships with an educator and/or social worker, could learn about these problems prior to the examination. The expertise of the educator and social worker and/or psychologist should then be incorporated as part of the low vision service to deal with these problems effectively.

Another area of the parent/child relationship that might interfere with the low vision rehabilitation process is denial by the parent that the impairment exists. For example, a child who had cataracts removed at age three received a prescriptive lens as well as other optical aids from a low vision specialist. A hearing aid was prescribed by another specialist to correct a hearing impairment. Significant improvement in performance was noted. However, his mother could not accept the appearance of both the aphakic prescription and hearing aids. She consistently removed the glasses and hearing aids only to render the child to his handicaps. A combined effort by the educator and social worker, in conjunction with a consultation with the low vision specialist, convinced the parent of the importance of the aids. This situation emphasizes again the need for a multidisciplinary approach in meeting the needs of the child. Without team effort and a holistic view of the child, such a misunderstanding on the part of the parent could have gravely affected the child's performance.

In dealing with both the overprotective parent and the parent who fails to accept the child's impairment, the optometrist must remain consistent in explanations about the impairment and low vision recommendations. The explanations should be brief and to the point. Medical and optical terminology should be explained in a language that the parents can understand. Too often, information given will be in excess of what the parent can comprehend at the time of the examination. Confusion may result. Also, a parent may leave the examination understanding the optometrist's explanation but experiencing feelings of personal guilt. This guilt may be projected as disappointment about the results of the examination.

The low vision specialist should be aware of these possibilities and be ready to deal with them. A telephone call to the parent a week or so after the examination may uncover some of these problems. A follow-up explanation may be effective in eliminating any misunderstanding, or in the case of defensive projections, counseling for the parent and/or the child might be recommended.

Considering the Classroom and Home Environment
Before prescribing optical aids and devices for the school-age child, the practitioner needs to know how the child functions in the classroom and at home. The educator may be willing to offer this information in a brief report. There are standard functional low vision assessment instruments available. However, a more informal approach may suffice by simply discussing with the educator the type of information that is needed. For example, the optometrist will benefit from information about where the child is seated in the classroom, where the windows are located, whether glare from the windows presents any particular problems, and what the lighting is like in the classroom. Optical aids may be totally ineffective if glare or inadequate lighting interferes with the child's ability to use them.

Information concerning how the child uses his vision in the habitual environment may enable the optometrist to be more precise in the examination. For example, does the child turn his head to one side when viewing at near or at distance, squint when looking at a distance, cover one eye when reading, point to the material being read or lose his place frequently while reading. Head turns or covering one eye may be an indication of difficulty with binocular alignment, while squinting may indicate an uncorrected refractive error. Loss of place while reading may indicate functional difficulties of fixations, pursuits and/or saccades.

Information about the child's coordination, balance and spatial organization will enable the optometrist to understand how the child uses peripheral vision to match information with motor movement and orientation. Knowing that the child consistently bumps into objects on one side or trips over objects will give the optometrist reason to consider a possible field loss prior to the examination. Regarding personal hygiene and appearance, the child who fails to comb his hair may not be able to see himself in the mirror. This need would be considered in the low vision examination.

The most important consideration is why this child is being referred for a low vision examination. The educator should discuss what specific function needs to be improved. The answer to this and other information mentioned above may save a considerable amount of time during the examination.

Reporting to the Educator

The concept of a low vision service is only as good as the communication between the professionals involved. The very best low vision examination can be diminished in quality if the educator and/or parents do not understand the implications of the examination or how the child is to use the aids.

One educator thought that the cap that snapped onto the front of her student's hand-held telescope was a dust cover. Two years after the examination, she learned that it was a reading cap. When the child used the telescope with the cap, both teacher and pupil were surprised to find that reading could be performed at an intermediate range. While both were elated to think that the device could be used to view intermediate ranges, it was unfortunate that two years had lapsed without the child benefiting from the prescribed cap.

The low vision specialist must provide basic information concerning the diagnosis and etiology in language that is easily understood. Acuity measurements for both distance and near ranges should be stated along with testing distance. It may be beneficial to include both uncorrected and best corrected measurements. Field measurements for distance (if taken) and for near should be given with an explanation of how they may affect the child's performance. Refractive findings should be included with a brief discussion, if appropriate, about the type of prescription given and whether contact lenses were prescribed or considered.

A discussion of the child's binocular state and how the visual condition may or may not contribute to fatigue levels, loss of attention, and reading difficulty may be helpful to the educator.

The improved acuity measurements and an explanation of how they are to be used should be provided along with the aids prescribed. The optometrist should mention any difficulties the child had in using the aid and should suggest, if appropriate, how the educator may effectively assist in training the child. Print size should be discussed. A range of print sizes rather than just one should be offered. The educator may find that the child will work more effectively with certain types of print, depending on the child's fatigue level, lighting, or subject covered. A final statement should include a recommendation for a follow-up visit.

By communicating with the educator, the low vision specialist can help to insure that the recommendations from the examination will be followed. Also, if a problem develops, such as a misunderstanding about the use of the aids, the report can answer many questions.

Summary
The low vision specialist must recognize that the examination of a child should include an analysis of function and performance. Further, the needs of the child must be evaluated with a developmen-

tal understanding and with a qualitative analysis of vision. The traditional quantitative means of vision assessment may be of limited effectiveness if used as the sole means for prescriptive determination.

Early intervention is the key to effectively dealing with the unique difficulties of each child and the negative effects of social pressures. Also, early intervention is the best means for affecting the overall development of the child. The recognition by the optometrist of the dynamic relationship of vision to function and development will enable the practitioner to apply traditional prescriptive techniques to low vision care to meet developmental needs of the child. The success of the low vision examination should not be measured by the improvement in the child's acuity through use of the aids, but rather by the improvement in the child's performance in his habitual environments.

The challenge of providing low vision services for a child is one in which the low vision specialist must recognize that his effectiveness can be maximized by utilizing the skills of other professionals. Thus, the concept of a multidisciplinary service can be developed only when all professionals communicate and work toward the common goal of meeting the needs of the child.

Educational Programs for the Visually Impaired Child

The setting for the education of the visually impaired may vary. This largely depends on the program set up by the state or town and can be influenced by the population of visually impaired children for whom a city or town must provide services. One means by which a visually handicapped child receives special education is by attending a school for the blind. Such a school has a staff of specially trained teachers and orientation and mobility instruction for the visually impaired. Schools for the blind are usually residential, with the children going home on weekends. In some instances, children are transported to such schools on a daily basis.

The resource room is another place where the special needs of the visually impaired child are met. The resource room is usually housed within a regular public school, and a teacher for the visually impaired is employed to provide special services. The visually impaired children are transported from throughout the town or district on a daily basis. The objective of the resource room is to program children into everyday classroom settings with non-visually impaired children. This is known as mainstreaming. The amount of time the visually impaired child is mainstreamed is dependent upon the amount of individualized support service the child needs from the resource teacher. In the resource room the child is instructed in specialized curricula areas and in the use of various adaptive devices. The number of resource rooms that a school district will establish is determined by the population of visually impaired children for whom it must provide special services.

A third means by which the visually impaired child can receive special educational services is through the itinerant teacher program. Where such a program exists, the visually impaired child attends his neighborhood school and is an integral part of the regular school day. The teacher for the visually impaired travels from school to school to serve the visually impaired child in the classroom where he has been assigned. The regular classroom teacher can expect to receive assistance and consultation from the itinerant teacher, who will also schedule direct tutorial services for the visually mpaired child. If a child cannot attend his neighborhood school due to another type of physical impairment or learning disability, the itinerant teacher will travel to wherever the child is assigned.

CHAPTER XI

THE MULTIHANDICAPPED CHILD

The child with motor impairments in addition to visual impairment has complex functional and habilitative needs. As described in the chapter about development and vision, the learning experience of a child with a motor impairment is limited, sometimes severely, because information cannot be matched accurately between motor and senses. The impairment often affects speech patterns, visual discrimination, movement, balance, posture and sensory discrimination. Having to deal with a motor impairment as well as a sight impairment often causes medical and educational professionals to overlook the often serious visual difficulty.

A sight and a vision impairment has been called "the hidden handicap" because in most instances it cannot be seen. On the other hand, a motor impairment like a deformed limb, abnormal posture, muscular spasms or hypotonic muscle tone is more obvious. While it is with good intentions, professionals and lay persons usually treat the motor impairment as soon as possible with medical and therapeutic techniques. Progress in educational and habilitative therapy is often limited because the sight and/or vision impairment is not treated at the same time.

Unfortunately, most multihandicapped children do not receive appropriate vision services until they are of school age and particular problems with visual discrimination are observed. The exception is when a child has a strabismus, and the eye turn is visible. Referrals will often be made for the consideration of surgery. While this at least enables the child to have an eye examination, this form of treatment often does not consider the relationship of visual function and performance to the overall neuro-motor and functional abilities of the child.

Previous discussions have emphasized that the motor system provides a base for visual function. It is critical that the motor-impaired child be evaluated not only in terms of eye health, ocular motility and alignment, but also with regard to the functional relationship between the visual and neuro-motor processes. The motor system, through the influences of the kinesthetic and proprioceptive systems, will affect how the child utilizes the visual process. This effect will take the form of variations in eye alignment, tracking ability, accommodative function, fixation abilities, and a variety of other functional behaviors.

Case Study

At the time of this study, Andrea was three years old and a cerebral palsy victim with motor spasticity. She demonstrated a right esotropia and an inability to track and fixate when she was placed in a sitting position. While in the seated position her head and neck flexed and motor tone increased. When placed on her back on a mat and with her pelvis lifted onto the examiner's knees, tracking patterns as well as alignment of the eyes improved.

The postural change affected Andrea's functional use of vision. This case study demonstrates that the motor system does influence visual function. It particularly shows that stress in the neuro-motor system will affect eye alignment and ocular motility. Sensory function of the visual system can be limited as well.

Developing a model of vision that incorporates the neuro-motor system as the base for visual function enables us to understand how motor spasticity and imbalances in the neuro-motor system can interfere with visual performance, and vice versa. It is imperative, therefore, that the multihandicapped child be examined in a variety of positions to observe the effect of the neuro-motor state on the visual system. When possible, the therapist, occupational and/or physical, should assist the optometrist or ophthalmologist in discussing the motor impairment and determining the appropriate positioning for the child. The following discussion will offer some guidelines for evaluating the multihandicapped child. As there will always be individual exceptions, these must be utilized as guides.

Examination Procedure:

When introduced to the child, the examiner should first observe whether there are neuro-motor flexion or extension patterns. (Flexion means that the child is leaning forward, typically with his head down and tucked to the chest. In the extension posture the child is positioned with head back and arms out. Hypotonic (low) muscle tone or hypertonic (spastic) muscle tone can occur in either states of flexion or extension. Secondly, the examiner should note if the child is leaning to one side, indicating a possible imbalance due to a right- or left-side weakness. Also, the examiner should review the type of chair, head supports or other prosthetics that may affect his posture and in turn affect vision. If the child is ambulatory, the examiner should observe the child standing and walking. When the child is able to stand on two feet, previously observed motor patterns may change. Bearing weight on the feet may cause a child who was in flexion pattern in a seated position to show extension postures or weight shifting to the right or left side while standing.

Head position is very important. The examiner should continually observe whether the head is rotated differently in standing or walking postures than in sitting postures. Also, if the head assumes a state of extension or flexion differently than what was observed with overall muscle tone in the body, it should be noted.

If possible, a thorough history should be taken with the parent, therapist and educator accompanying the child. Information concerning the birth or any traumas incurred as well as medical treatment and medications should be reviewed. If the child has had any seizures, that information should be included with dates of occurrence. When the history reveals active seizures, the examiner should take caution not to flash lights directly into the eyes of the child since flashing lights, or even stimulation from a penlight turned on and off repeatedly, have been known to initiate seizures.

The examiner should then complete a thorough ocular health assessment including external and internal evaluation of the eyes. If nystagmus (a constant jerk of both eyes simultaneously caused by neurological problems) is present, a thorough evaluation should be made in the cardinal positions of gaze while the child fixates on an object. The nystagmus should also be evaluated when posture is varied, such as when the child is lying on his back or on his side. Changes in position that influence the vestibular and kinesthetic systems will sometimes change the amount of nystagmus. This is common in children with cerebral palsy. Often when the child lies on his back or side, nystagmus subsides and fixation abilities can improve.

A cover test in a variety of positions should be performed to evaluate eye alignment. Changes in kinesthetic and vestibular stimulation will often affect eye alignment. Not only should strabismus be evaluated, but the examiner should pay attention to states of phoria. The convergence ability of the child should be assessed. For young children or those low in functioning, an interesting accommodative stimulus should be used. Not only should the quantity or extent to which they are able to converge and maintain eye alignment be assessed, but the quality of their performance should be evaluated as well. That is, does the child work hard at converging his eyes, and does the examiner observe frequent fixation losses and an inability to sustain fixation on an object?

A thorough refraction using trial lenses and retinoscopy should be performed. Since the voropter will affect the child's posture and position, it should not be used. Variations in posture will also affect the refraction. It is important that the child be placed in a position that is comfortable and supportive. A reclining position on a mat provides support and can enable the examiner to perform the refraction effectively. If the child is spastic, he needs to be supported with pillows or rolls so that his legs are not left suspended, and that support to the back and neck is complete.

A near refraction should be performed after the distance refractive state has been analyzed. With the refractive corrections in place, the near refraction may be done while the child fixates on a small silver bell, a hand-held puppet, or another visually stimulating object. The near refraction should analyze whether accommodative (focusing) states are equal and balanced for the two eyes. In addition, the grasp and release of accommodation and how easily accommodation is sustained to the plane of regard again must be assessed. The near refraction should always be done in varying postures and fixations to different points of focus. When accommodation lags or varies, plus lenses are to be introduced, and changes in fixation and accommodation evaluated.

When possible, touch-point (reaching and touching) activities can be used and accuracy measured. Touch-point activities should be performed with and without the distance prescription and again with plus lenses or those lenses found to be most effective in improving accommodation function.

Information about eye alignment, convergence ability, fixation and tracking should be analyzed in a manner that allows the examiner to functionally assess the patient's abilities as well as to develop a means for visual rehabilitation. It is extremely important to provide information to parents, educators and therapists with regard to compensations for visual inabilities that the child must make. For example, the child with a right esotropia who attempts to establish binocularity may turn his head to the right. Materials presented to the left of the child's midline will be in a field of lesser demand, enabling the child better alignment of the head and neck. This will affect the child's balance and will further support the child in reaching and eye-hand coordination. Unfortunately, the examiner often overlooks the opportunity to provide this information, which, in addition to improving the child's functional ability, will also establish the credibility for the optometrist with the parents.

A retinoscopy with trial lenses and a trial frame should be included in the examination. As stated before, a voropter is an inappropriate instrument to use to determine the appropriate lens prescription. Although trial lenses require more time and expertise, a more accurate prescription can be produced. In situations where the child responds negatively to trial lenses, radical retinoscopy can be used. In this procedure the optometrist varies his working distance and uses the reciprocal working distance when the neutral reflex is measured to determine the power of the refractive state. For the exact technique, the reader should review other sources mentioned in the reference section of this book (Borish, 1970).

Near retinoscopy should be performed before and after distance retinoscopic findings. Often children who have motor and neurological impairments will show imbalances in accommodative abilities. Unless this is treated, the ability of a child to function at a near range will be greatly interfered with. The examiner should add plus lenses to distance retinoscopic findings until a balanced near finding is achieved. The examiner should do this despite the fact that one eye may accept +2.00 addition and the other eye +0.75 addition. The goal is to achieve balance in the visual system.

Balance in the visual system must be understood with respect to the motor and neurological imbalances that affect autonomic function. Imbalances in motor and neurological function of the central nervous system can cause stress, affecting the autonomic nervous system, thus altering the accommodative response. Conversely, by utilizing lenses that reduce visual stress, it is not uncommon to observe postural changes. A confrontation visual field test may be effective in analyzing the scope of field. Children who have cortical visual impairment often also have a visual field loss. The visual field loss may interfere with the ability to relate the ambient process of vision to postural adjustments. For example, a child with a right homonymous hemianopsia (right field loss) will often neglect his right side. Since the child does not see in the right field of gaze, he places visual emphasis on motor functions on the left side. The neglect to the right side may interfere with handedness, posture, and balance while seated and walking.

Visual field testing may require two individuals. One is seated in front of the child who is playing with a toy, attempting to gain fixation. The other individual, seated behind the child, introduces a penlight or other stimulating object in a peripheral arc from behind the child to the front midline. By patching one eye, the monocular visual field can be evaluated. The individual seated in front of the child must monitor the child's eye position. When the child first sees the penlight through peripheral awareness, he will often make a fixation change from the toy to the penlight. A rough approximation in degree or scope of field can be made by the person seated in front of the child.

Often visual field testing and visual acuity testing cannot be completed during the limited time of the in-office examination. It is important for therapists, parents and educators to follow through at home or in school in order to average information over a period of time. Parents, therapists and educators should be encouraged to perform these tests and bring findings to follow-up visits. The examiner will then be able to spend more time in other areas of testing and treatment to improve relationships among vision, motor and balance processes.

Upon completion of this assessment, the examiner should work with appropriate lenses and prisms in an attempt to establish greater balance of visual and motor functions. The examiner should seek information from the occupational and physical therapists regarding the child's motor abilities. Since the motor system provides the basis by which ocular alignment and visual skills are established, it is important to evaluate the child in a position that will offer the least stress to the central nervous system. If the clinician has limited understanding of cerebral dysfunctions that cause cerebral palsy, muscular dystrophy, etc., he should consult with the physical and/or occupational therapist to learn about the neuro-motor dysfunction. Generally, seating a child upright in a chair that does not support the child's pelvis or thoracic area may cause stress and increase motor spasticity. This can affect visual functions and cause ocular malalignment, accommodative imbalances and/or spasms. The spastic child needs an appropriate seat that offers support. The best position for a young child may be lying on his back on a mat with legs flexed up onto the examiner's thighs. In this way the pelvis is extended in the posterior portion with flexion in the abdominal area. Also, a small roll may be placed under the neck to support the head.

Examination of the spastic child in this position often will show visual states that are completely different than those taken when the child is seated or standing. Another effective position in stabilizing the visual state is to roll the child onto his side while supporting the neck with a roll or pillow. The kinesthetic, vestibular, and tactual stimulation that he receives in this position may also reinforce visual functions. The clinician may find that fixation, tracking and convergence abilities may improve considerably.

For the child with hypotonic or low tone in his neuro-motor system, posture must be supported so the head does not dangle to the side or in front. Whatever support necessary to reduce stress in the neuro-motor system should be provided. This includes holding the child or supporting his head and neck with rolls or pillows so that stress is not induced. Another position that is effective in examining the hypotonic child is to have the child lie on his stomach over a large ball or a cylindrical roll that supports the child on the midline of the body. This kinesthetic and tactual stimulation on the midline will help the child organize central nervous system responses. This may affect visual functions, thus enabling the child to have improved fixations on the midline.

Emphasis must be placed on the support of the central nervous system and the reduction of stress throughout the neuro-motor system in the examination of the multihandicapped child. When this is achieved, the visual state may be analyzed with the least interference from either spastic or low-tone conditions. This cannot be understated. The behavioral analysis must be continued utilizing lens and prism combinations.

The discussion of various neuro-motor states will be dealt with in another chapter. However, it is important to emphasize here that the examiner must recognize that these conditions interfere with visual function, and very often visual states will reinforce and even cause conditions of flexion and extension patterns. The examination of the multihandicapped child should not end at the point of correction of refractive states. The examiner must understand that the child's performance depends upon his ability to differentiate neuro-motor functions as well as visual perception. When there is difficulty differentiating motor movements and organization within the central nervous system, the child will have difficulty in his ability to fixate and track. The converse is also true. When visual states interfere with ability to organize information, the child's ability to extend this organization to other sensory-motor processes will be affected. If visual stress can be reduced, it will have a positive effect on the differentiation of motor responses.

The examiner should observe postural shifts or adjustments that may be related to ocular alignment. If a child has an esotropia or an exotropia that is either congenital or post-surgically induced, appropriate compensation with yoked prisms may be considered. For example, if the child has a right esotropia and he is attempting to achieve binocularity, he may turn his head to the right. The head turn and the esotropia will often cause a midline shift due to the visual oculomotor imbalance. This midline shift will affect his ability to posture himself properly, in turn affecting other motor functions such as reaching or walking.

After the refraction and evaluation have been completed, the clinician may decide to work with yoked prisms. In the case above, yoked prisms with base-right orientation would be appropriate. Prisms of equal power would be added to each eye and would be placed with base-out for the right eye and base-in for the left eye. The prism would essentially shift the visual field over to the child's left side. This is the area that offers the least demand on the child's vision. If the child has attempted to turn his head to the right, essentially he has tried to posture the visual world to his left. The base-right yoked prism will accomplish the same by shifting his visual world to the left. This may cause a change in postural adjustment. The child may align his head more directly on midline because he does not have to compensate for oculomotor imbalances. Shifting the head to the midline will affect posture in the neck and shoulder areas. Often multihandicapped children with this type of oculomotor compensation and postural shifts will have spastic or fixed tone in the neck or shoulder areas. This fixed tone is often due to the compensations of visual imbalances. The base-right prism can stabilize and reduce stress in the vision, thereby reducing the state of muscle tension in the neck or shoulder area. In addition, there are other spatial effects from utilizing yoked prisms that will often cause postural changes due to a variation in the transfer of weight from one side to another.

The child with a bilateral esotropia will often exhibit postural imbalances of a more severe nature. The young multihandicapped child without the ability to align both eyes will attempt to posture the visual world in an area of least demand on his vision. For example, the child will often show extension of the head and neck. He will tip his head back, attempting to posture the visual world below his line of sight. For the multihandicapped child this can cause a hypertonic situation in the head, neck and shoulder areas. In turn, an inability to accurately negotiate upper-arm movements develops. Usually this fixed tone is dealt with through physical or occupational therapy. However, it must be recognized that this condition is often the result of stress in the visual system. By placing base- up yoked prisms of equal power before each eye, the visual world will be shifted downward or into an inferior position of gaze. The child will not have to extend his neck and head backward and in turn the visual field, being shifted to an area of lesser visual demand, will often produce a situation of decreased head extension and increased capital flexion. This is a more normal posture. In addition, another behavioral symptom of this condition are deep wrinkles and lines in the forehead. Because the child is unable to circumduct or elevate the two eyes together by manipulation of the superior rectus muscles, effort by the child to elevate the eyes is referred to the frontalis muscle. As the frontalis muscle contracts, deep furrows are formed in the forehead.

Further indication that the hypertonic condition in the neck and shoulder areas can cause spasticity in the frontalis muscle can be understood by studying anatomy of the head and neck. The frontalis muscle is connected to the galea aponeurotica, a thin tissue that extends from the frontalis muscle over the skull to the trapezius muscle in the neck. As the frontalis muscle contracts and pulls on the galea aponeurotica, tension will be created in the trapezius and neck muscles, causing high muscle tone in the neck and shoulder area.

Bilateral esotropia will also interfere with the child's ability to stand and walk because with the head in extension and the hypertonic condition in the neck and shoulder area, the midline is shifted to the posterior portion of the body. When the child attempts to bear weight on the feet, there may be an overcompensation due to the shift of midline posteriorly. This may in turn cause the child to lose balance, thereby interfering with the ability to stand or walk. Base-up yoked prisms may be effective in changing the visual-motor orientation, thereby affecting neuro-motor functions.

CHAPTER XII

POSITIONING ASPECTS OF SUCCESSFUL VISUAL INTERVENTION

In this chapter we will examine the special needs of individuals who have disorders of the central nervous system that affect their control of posture and movement and, in a large number of cases, their functional vision. This is a population that generally has no clear injury to the eyes per se and yet may have great difficulty organizing the visual system to utilize information received from the environment. A "functional disorder" may be mentioned without being identified early on as a specific problem that could respond to intervention.

In the general population there are people, children as well as adults, who have physical problems that are unrelated to the functioning of their visual systems. They may have a coincidental problem with vision along with conditions, such as polio or dystrophy, that affect the muscular system or injuries to the physical structure. Another group of children and adults have well-defined neurological conditions such as hemiplegia due to stroke, in which there is a strong likelihood that the responses of the eyes will mirror the responses of the body. There are also many who do not demonstrate visual complications with such neurological conditions. On the other hand, homonymous hemianopsia may be the complication of a brain hemorrhage or infection without any clear physical manifestations in that individual that affect posture and movement.

Neurological disorders that exist from birth or occur as the result of accident or illness are seldom as clearly defined as an adult hemiplegia, as they are not due to a limited area of the brain being affected but rather to developmental dysfunction. Children who have had problems since birth or an early age have never known the clear automatic feedback of normal postural control against gravity. In those cases the central nervous system fails to perform its function of coordinating control of the body and thus alters the functional base of all sensory systems. The fundamental movement patterns of the eyes have no base from which to mature, and there is a lack of synchrony between eyes and body.

Conscientious evaluation is not easy. These children may have had more than the average number of disagreeable experiences with professionals, merely because of their need for more than average amounts of medical care. As infants and young children, they overhear comments that they don't understand and are often handled in ways that are more efficient than sensitive. The similarity of any examination to these previous experiences may be a disadvantage to the optometrist. The ability to relate to the child beyond the disability will be a great strength. The fact that the small child can remain with his mother while responding to the optometrist also aids in establishing rapport. Brain-injured adults may also arrive in a very frustrated and depressed state, as many services offer diagnosis and general supervision rather than intervention that changes their functional state.

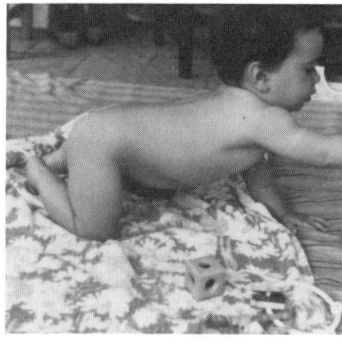
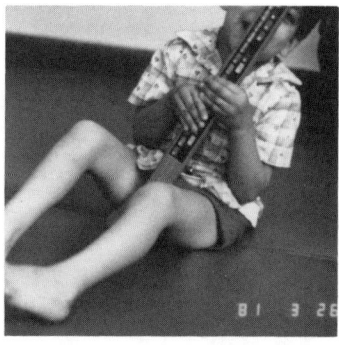

I. Normal posture. Normal posture control balances stability with mobility.

J. Abnormal posture. Excessive flexor tonus moves the center of gravity back and prevents comfortable floor sitting.

Complete examination of any functional system requires that we take into account the lack of developmental experience available to that system. When we are considering the interaction of postural control, movement and vision, a child's seemingly simple play activity becomes complex. Dysfunction in any one of these systems or limitations in their intracommunication results in poor organization of environmental impressions. Children with cerebral palsy may have such inadequate postural reactions that they are dependent on another person or special equipment to position them against gravity. Movement may be disjointed and appear inappropriate to the task, even when the child understands clearly what needs to be done. When the message of the central nervous system is expressed in the form of inadequate postural and movement responses, all other systems must compensate to organize function. The visual system, due to its strength of relating directly to the environment, is one of the strongest sources of compensation. That means that the system learns to react in a way that maximizes the security of the person and delivers the best information about the environment.

As with substitute movement patterns, the compensatory efforts of the visual system reach their maximum effectiveness and then begin to interfere with further maturation. Adaptations that should be relegated to the automatic level stay at consciousness and interfere with new learning. Children with high postural tone or spasticity typically rely on total patterns of movement and may use eye movement upward to initiate extension. Relaxation of the eyes, then, reduces the high tonus and lets the head fall forward into gravity. The child who lacks postural control may have random, in-

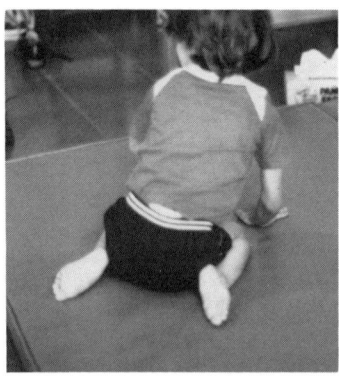
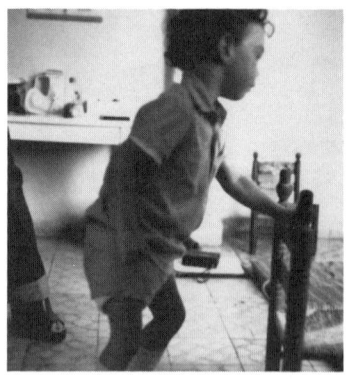

K. Sitting between legs. Sitting between the legs is to be avoided because it blocks active trunk adjustments for balance.

L. Poor control and high tone. High tonus limits normal sensory feedback and distorts the child's learning of movement.

appropriate movement of the eyes that mirrors the lack of postural control in his body.

A functional orientation to the visual examination is essential for any person who has a neurological disability. Aside from the fact that it requires ingenuity and creativity to analyze the relationship between the visual system and behavior, these individuals will require even more specialized observations. In some instances the child is able to move his eyes without an ability to direct vision intentionally. This is comparable to extraneous movement sometimes seen in the physical body. In the experience of very low postural tone or a basic inability to move the body, the child may capitalize on his control of eye movement. This type of child will use his eyes as a major form of communication, focusing repeatedly on what he wants or in the direction in which he wishes to be moved. Speech pathologists can capitalize on such reliable control of vision to fashion visual communication systems for the child who is unable to speak.

To evaluate the functional state of the visual system, it is most important to know whether head movement is possible in all directions and to the fullest potential range of movement. Without free excursion of the head, there may be a limited visual field used. In some cases the eyes are able to compensate by use of extreme movements. In those cases there may be problems of focusing, poor conjugate vision, or visual stress due to the effort at compensation.

Parents can offer essential information to help us understand their children. In cases of acquired brain injury the family can offer much information about the personality prior to the accident or illness, although that information is better acquired after the professional has demonstrated some ability to make a functional difference for the client. Parents will know or can observe whether the direction of the child's gaze correlates with the direction of the window from his crib. They can describe changes in head position when the child attempts a visual task or under which circumstances he loses interest in visual activity. When responding to a visual stimulus, the child may notably increase his postural tone. It is helpful perhaps

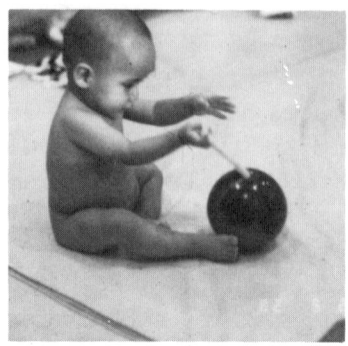 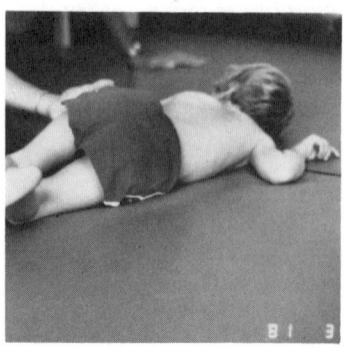

M. Normal fixing to focus. For the normal baby visual focus is a skill closely integrated with movement.

N. High tone moving. This boy has high intelligence but is unable to move his body in the way he knows it should move.

to think of this as an abnormal exaggeration of the postural fixation observed in the young infant when he needs to sustain visual focus for examination of some intriguing aspect of the environment.

It is always important to recognize that the nature of abnormal tonus is such that the individual each time associates it more closely with functional activity until the functional response does not occur without the tonus change and the abnormal tonus interferes with function. In the case of young children there is little or no normal sensory information to balance the abnormal, and consequently the child becomes more limited over time. We might think of the behavioral manifestations of the original disorder as increasing, although the brain dysfunction per se is a stable condition.

When assessing the outcome potential of a central nervous system disorder we are trying to anticipate the compensatory skill of that total system to use alternate pathways and synaptic connections to substitute for the ones that have been injured or rendered dysfunctional. The compensatory ability of the central nervous system has been well documented with adults. Bach-y-Rita (1980), a research neurologist, relates the story of his own father who suffered a severe stroke and made a complete physical, mental, and emotional recovery to full function. Years later, when he died of an unrelated cause, an autopsy revealed that one complete brain hemisphere had completely atrophied at the time of the hemorrhage and had remained that way for ten years, even though full function had returned. Young adults have remained in a coma for six months to one year, and two years after that were attending classes in a community college. These possibilities are mentioned for the benefit of clinicians who may be uncertain whether to follow their intuition to offer visual support for the traumatized child or adult who struggles to make a comeback.

Abnormal Postural Behavior

In the presence of abnormal postural behavior, a lack of movement of the body away from the surface is an overriding influence. The proprioceptive system is not able to coordinate these responses, and therefore effort on the part of the child to readapt the posture of the body results in total extensor responses or reflexive patterns that do not support body function. Attempts to use the sensory systems to gather information about the environment are thwarted by the energy lost in efforts to control posture.

The following premises are useful in the analysis of the reactions of a child, taking into account the personal history, the family experiences, observations of visual behavior, and the personality of the individual.

1. If a healthy adult is unable to move the child's body into a given position, the child will be unable to assume that position independently. This seems a simple premise until one observes that we frequently ask a child to reach for an object or keep his head in a given position without ever trying to place the body part ourselves. Willingness to touch the affected individual and move a body part gently will reveal much about the amount of effort used by that person to make the simplest response. It may be impossible for the individual to control movement of the limbs in a predictable way. Eye blinks are often the most basic communication initiated by the individual and may be used to answer yes/no questions.

2. If we introduce or superimpose movement of a body part that consequently threatens balance or causes a total reaction of another part of the body, the person with brain dysfunction will intuitively

avoid the first movement. This does not mean that he is unable to coordinate the movement, only that he cannot handle the consequences. As movement potential becomes chronically limited in range and diversity, the child loses ability to perform the avoided movement and substitutes abnormal reactions in order to function. This is somewhat analogous to the physical atrophy that occurs in situations of limited use of a body part over time.

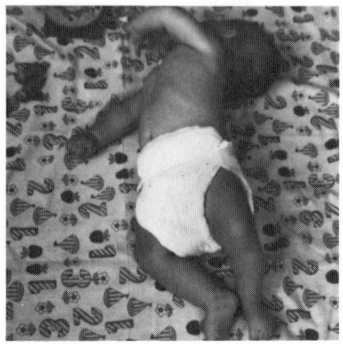

O. Abnormal posture with visual focus. Vision will lead postural adaptation even when the responses are abnormal.

3. If the head cannot be stabilized with normal control, the eyes will not be able to function in a normal, automatic and effortless way. There will be some attempt to compensate as the child begins to use existing vision: the head may be fixed to one side or tipped back in a slightly extended posture, causing an apparent shortening of the neck. It will be helpful here to attempt to bring the head forward to feel the resistance and in some cases to ask the child to close his eyes while his head is brought forward. When the head can be brought forward with gentle assistance, there is less likely to be significant structural limitation, and the child is a good candidate for effective use of prism lenses. While informed use of prism lenses can make dramatic alterations in postural adjustment by changing the environmental information that affects balance, the structure must be free to respond to these new messages. In this regard it is vital that the optometrist and the therapist work closely together. Prism lenses, especially base-up, have been dramatic in changing the strong tonus in the flexor surface of the body that pulls a child into gravity. In other sections of this book the interested reader can learn more of the criteria for determining individual recommendations. Behavioral change and postural adaptation are the best monitors of successful change.

4. If there is no point of stable alignment, normal or abnormal, for the neck and head, there is no physiological base from which the eye muscles can organize their movement. This lack of stable alignment will result in a lack of postural control for the neck and consequently the eyes. There will be a tendency to scan with the eyes without the ability to control fixation or, consequently, to develop essential eye-hand coordination. Assisting the child by stabilizing the neck externally will aid the organization of physical movement for the eyes. This may be done simply with a towel rolled lengthwise and placed firmly in a position like that of a fur collar. It may be helpful to think of this as a temporary facilitation of eye movements that have not previously been used in order to stimulate use of the visual system, particularly for the multihandicapped child who has few resources and for whom we need to demonstrate some sign of constructive intellectual activity. As better eye movement permits the visual system to mature in its function, such external supports may be reduced.

5. High extensor tonus of the neck tends to be associated with upward movements of the eyes. The backward movement of the head that results from this upward rolling of the eyes may be initiated either by an attempt to use the eyes or by an increase in extensor tonus in the back and the neck itself. Tonus distribution in extension is increased when the child rests on a firm support in a supine, or face up, position. When the same child learns to sit or is propped in a sitting position by artificial supports, there are likely to be secondary compensations in the form of increased tonus over the flexor surface of the body. Being threatened with the constant possibility of falling backward, the child may use whatever force he has to pull himself forward into flexion. This forward flexion may sometimes be mistaken as representing a benign collapse, when actually there is considerable force in the forward

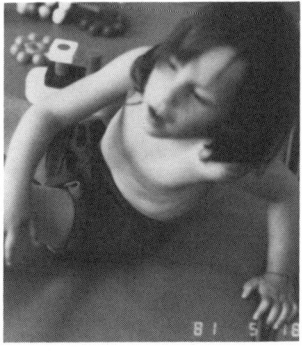

P. Sitting with symmetry. Lack of rotation in the trunk increases the effort needed for postural change.

movement, and the examiner will no doubt find it difficult to bring the child to an upright position. After several years of the abnormal adaptation, the vestibular system no longer differentiates the correct signals, and the body fails to support itself.

6. Avoidance of extension in the neck tends to be associated with keeping the eyes in a downward gaze. In this situation the eyes will assist the control of the body and avoid the takeover of extensor tonus, as described above. Bright children learn to do this early and may even appear to have a field loss or lack of awareness of visual stimuli above the horizontal midline. Movement of the eyes upward may result in a sudden loss of postural control, a frightening experience.

7. Lack of sensory awareness of one side of the body tends to be associated with less eye movement toward that side and/or less movement of the eye on that side. There may be less use of the eye on the more affected side to the point that acuity is actually affected. This is also influenced strongly by the body posture of the individual and takes into account the postural adaptations. The more affected side tends to be retracted, which creates a natural tendency to tilt the head toward the paper on the "better side" and use that eye more. In reality, there is no "better" or "worse" side, as the seemingly less-affected side of the body soon attempts to compensate and may actually become almost hyperkinetic in its attempt to take over functions of the less able parts. In therapeutic physical handling it is essential to inhibit constantly the overactive responses as the less active postural responses are encouraged. The reactions of the total body must be given consideration and the child helped to gain an experience of dynamic symmetry through careful handling combined with the proprioceptive firm pressure experience of weight- bearing. The adult must also be assisted to regain this sensation of postural symmetry, although the therapist will often work with the client in a seated posture in order to move in and out of a vertical midline orientation.

Physical Manifestations of Lack of Postural Control

Developmentally, it is useful to think of normal extension of the body against gravity as starting at the neck and moving to the head and then down the length of the spine. Early righting reactions are further integrated by the equilibrium reactions to form a subconscious network of control against the force of gravity. Normally, we give no conscious thought to these reactions and are consequently free to put our attention on communication, creative thoughts, or concentrated intellectual pursuit. Our subconscious network of righting and equilibrium reactions should be available as needed to protect us and to stimulate movement against gravity. It is a fundamental concept that when a body part or functional system, such as vision, is involved in maintaining a body position, that same part or system is not available to perform its own specific function.

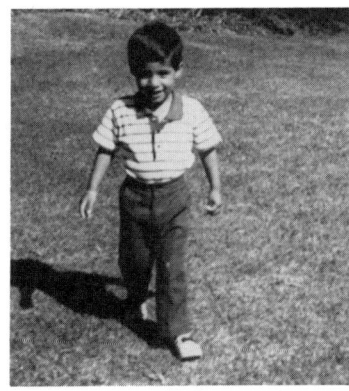

Q. Skilled movement. To achieve control in an upright alignment requires preparation of many postural components.

Poor head control is probably the most significant physical limitation since it affects the entire body and the effective use of the sensory systems. There will often be a sharp contrast between use of the eyes in a supported position and in independent sitting, for example. This also occurs with the use of the hands, another peripheral task of coordination. It would be useful to offer more support to the child in the upright position instead of having him struggle to maintain his alignment so that he has no energy left for fine coordination, especially that of eyes and hands. To offer a meaningful service to such children, the therapist must be prepared to help in the organization of the postural base and the teacher to consider postural needs in the classroom.

Chronic posturing of the head may be due to malalignment of the cervical spine or lack of balance and muscle action, as well as a lack of balance in the use of the eyes. It is often apparent in casual observation of the child in the waiting area or in general visual tasks designed to put the child at ease. In the case of children who spend much of their school day strapped into special chairs, it is important to know whether the child usually has the option of moving his head for visual adjustment. Such a child may be dependent on positioning by the teacher, classroom aide or one of his physically mobile peers.

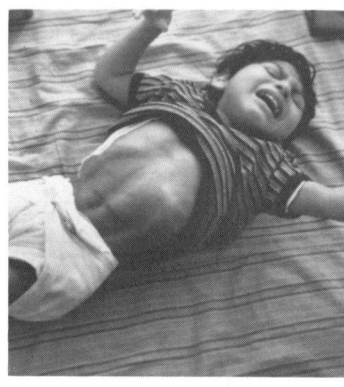

R. Severely involved child--multihandicapped. Significant neuromotor disability without treatment becomes more severe due to lack of movement experience.

A lack of trunk control is often characterized by seemingly erratic tilting to one side and then to another. This will include movements of the head that attempt to stabilize the trunk. Use of vision will be adversely affected by poorly designed straps or supports that compromise free movement of the diaphragm or the proper alignment of the spine. Poor correlation between trunk and head positions becomes chronic and limits the functioning of vision, vestibular reactions, and hearing, as well as the expression of fine coordination skill. The first line of intervention should be restoration of the structural alignment to stimulate optimal development. This suggests professional coordination between the therapist, optometrist, classroom teacher and the parents.

Poor control of limb movement may be general or concentrated in the upper or lower extremities or on one side of the body. A general problem may be reflected in inadequate trunk control, while disturbed coordination of the arms and hands may originate in a lack of stability or excessive tension of the shoulders. The latter may start with alignment problems of the spinal column or lack of

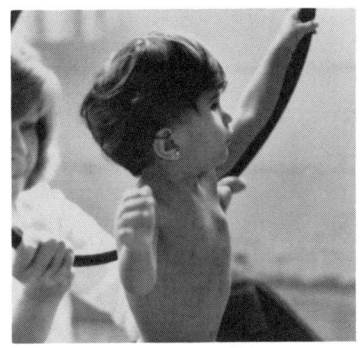 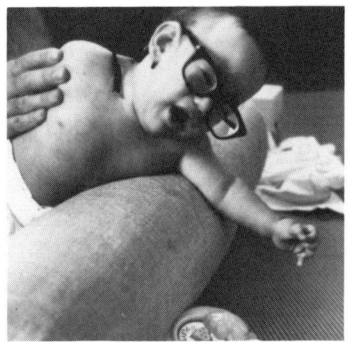

S. *Active treatment. An active response on the part of the child is useful after adequate preparation in treatment.*

developmental activation of the shoulders in infancy. There tends to be an inverse relationship between trunk tone and postural tone in the limbs, so offering more adequate support to the trunk often eases the struggle against gravity and normalizes the postural tone. In the case of chronic reactions in older children it will be necessary to offer direct treatment experiences during which the child can experience a more normal dynamic alignment and the possibility of movement without such excessive effort. Quality movement responses proceed from well- aligned postures that are ready to change according to our needs.

Incoordination of righting and equilibrium reactions is generally accompanied by problems of postural tonus. As the vestibular system is so closely aligned in its structure and its function with the visual system, there will usually be an attempt by the visual system to support posture against gravity. This fatigues the visual system over time and leaves it without the necessary experience of focusing the eyes with the hands. Since righting reactions

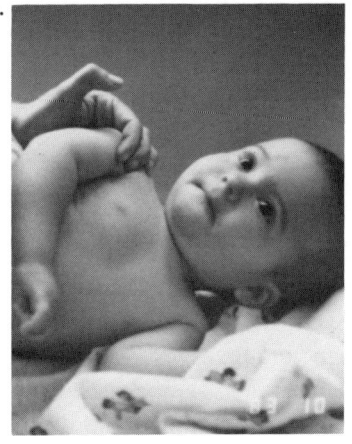

T. *Therapy. The therapist gives the child the sensation of normal movement patterns that he has not achieved independently.*

represent a fundamental coping with the influence of gravity, their lack of expression results in lack of movement. Equilibrium responses can be excessive in their expression when there is an imbalance within the proprioceptive system, with the vestibular input being stronger than that of the deep pressure receptors. Persons with that condition tend to flail their limbs and use excessive movement in tasks that require precision. Offering some compression to the trunk with simple hand pressure over the shoulders will assist the organization of movement. This clinical situation is frequently referred to as "athetoid-like" in movement quality, and the personality of this person tends to be rather labile with strong fluctuations in response.

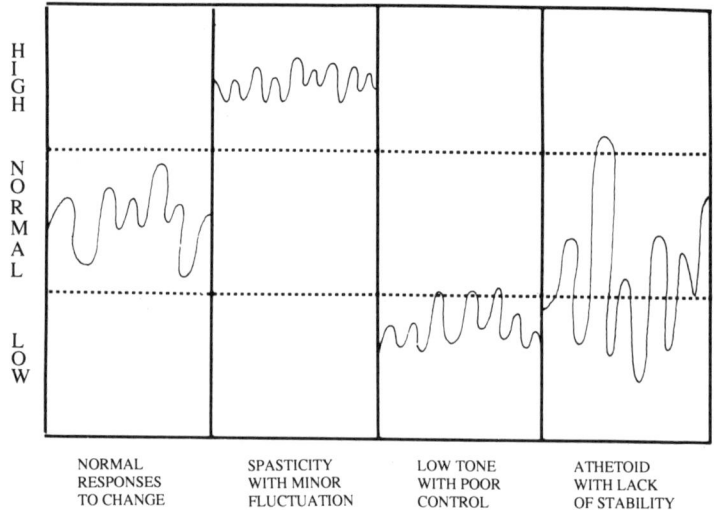

Figure 4. Normal and Abnormal Tonus

Normal postural tonus should fluctuate within a range adequate to support us against gravity and low enough to permit effortless movement. There is a readiness factor in normal tonus that supports us in our intention to move at any time, even with significant changes in speed, such as dashing to answer a telephone. High tonus limits the initiation of movement: there is a fear of postural change and a lack of balance reactions. The person tends to orient the body to a symmetrical position and seldom moves from that alignment. In such a situation the stimulation of lateral movement of the eyes could be an important contribution to change.

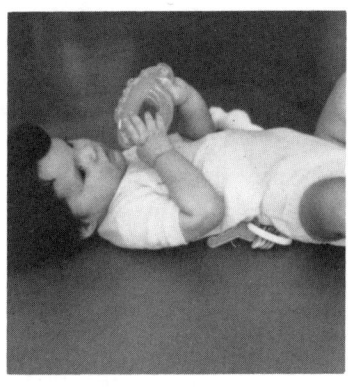

U. Baby with low tonus. Low postural tonus limits trunk movement, which is essential for good anti-gravity control, and visual experiences.

The contrasting situation, that of excessively low tonus, reduces the amount of movement as the body weight is pulled into gravity. The limbs may move to touch an object or to interact with an adult, but the proximal body associated with that limb remains fixed. Kicking of the legs, for example, is limited in excursion and, more importantly, is not accompanied by the lifting of the pelvis, which also activates the diaphragm. Consequently, the child with low tonus tends to have limited volume to his voice. Ironically, the child who demonstrates excessive high tone or spasticity initially may demonstrate low tone once the spasticity is reduced with therapeutic techniques. This is sometimes referred to as spasticity with a low tone base. It is a difficult problem for the therapist since the low tone must be stimulated to a normal level without exciting unwanted spasticity.

A fluctuation of tone is referred to as athetosis, from a Greek origin meaning "a lack of posture." The child tends to fix proximal parts of his own body in position in order to control his movement responses, although this consequently limits his range of movement and the development of graded control. These uncontrolled movement responses are also seen in some cases of multiple sclerosis and degenerative conditions of the central nervous system. While most experienced clinicians agree that there is a significant reduction in the number of pure athetoid individuals from birth as compared to 20 years ago, there are still persons struggling with movement patterns that fit the general description, so the term is useful to know.

Positioning the Client for Examination

When confronted with either an adult or a child who has sustained a brain injury, it is a good idea to note the postural characteristics: Is there an ability to sit independently, or is the person relying on another person or a protective chair? Does movement tend to be free or restricted? Is there some symmetry to the position of the body? Does the person initiate movement or rely on care givers?

Don't be fooled by the overly solicitous family member who takes charge. Try to establish some rapport directly with the client. Most commonly in the case of central nervous system disorders the person understands more than he can easily express. Often there is a delay in the mental processing of a request so that the person may answer several minutes later with an appropriate response. Be alert to this phenomenon, especially in the case of traumatic injuries.

After noting the initial posture, attempt to make a simple change to determine the resistance to movement or even to your touch. In the case of a child who is obviously more secure in his mother's arms, you might wish to check some responses of the visual system first and then attempt the movement. A friendly lifting of the arm or leg in play will tell you much about the relative weight of the limb and the changes in the body position as a result of the change in balance.

If the person accepts your touch, you will have no difficulty placing the palm of your hand behind his neck. At first, this may give you very little information, but soon your experience will suggest whether the tension that you feel is sufficient to prevent lifting the head forward or to limit lateral excursion of the head and the eyes. A finger placed lightly on the chest or the shoulder while the eyes move to follow your stimulus will be enough to sense the stiffening or increased tonus that tends to accompany visual activation. Knowing that this tension exists may suggest specific intervention at the visual level that might contribute to the lessening of the stress.

If the person is unable to turn his head to one side, it is a good idea to assist the movement. It is possible to feel whether there is a slow resistance throughout the range that suggests a neuromotor involvement with an increase in postural tone as opposed to an abrupt stop in the movement that can represent a structural limitation. Tracking tasks may be assisted by having the person turn his head to one side. Individuals who have postural problems that originated in infancy with the evolution of rotation of the body around the longitudinal axis will successfully track an object from one side to the other with the eyes to one side after being unable to perform the same task with the eyes forward. By turning the face to the side, we introduce a rotation component in the posture that frees the eyes to move in a more differentiated way.

When presenting a visual task to a person with poor control of his physical body, it is best to offer additional postural stability. This might be in the form of cushions, a different chair, or the physical assistance of the parent or family member. The objective is to observe whether the quality of the response improves with the additional support. This information may alter recommendations for lenses as well as suggestions for classroom placement and educational management. Trunk stability can usually be improved by aligning the shoulders directly over the hips. This will offer a better possibility for the arms to move and the head to align with the trunk.

Performance on two or three tasks can be compared with and without supplementary postural support in order to understand the interaction between postural control and visual system function for the individual. Priorities in treatment and education as well as direct visual intervention will become clearer as this information is gathered.

Alternative positions may be close to the original posture but take advantage of a different type of support, a new relationship to gravity, or a change in the surface texture. In cases of sensitivity to touch it is useful to realize that the central nervous system is calmed by firm pressure, smooth surfaces, and slow, predictable rhythms.

Light touch, rapid staccato contact, and irregular surfaces are excitatory and even noxious to some systems. The support of one's own weight tends to be organizing and may assist the child in making a visual response. The small child may like to be in a prone, tummy-lying position with a small roll of towel under his chest. An older individual might be brought forward to take weight on his elbows to change the postural alignment of the trunk. Providing a support for the back of the head in a seated position removes the stress from the back of the neck and may also change the movement potential of the eyes.

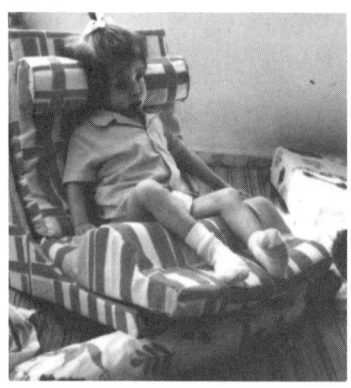

V. *Positioning in sitting. Seating supports should maintain the child's position without reliance on the straps used for safety.*

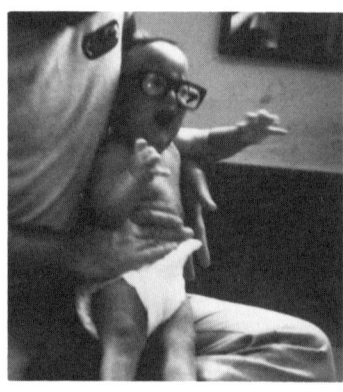

W. *Positioning. Crying increases tonus and makes it difficult to adapt the child's body to a new position.*

While many therapists have had no experience working with the visual system, most will be interested in the contributions that visual change can make in the physical functioning of their clients. Distractibility is often reduced. Increased awareness of the environment may motivate physical exploration. Specific reorientation of visual focus may even change the potential of an individual for independent ambulation. Changes in postural tone give the therapist greater possibilities for physical handling.

In exchange, the therapist who is trained in a neurodevelopmental approach or similar holistic view of the many aspects of neurological dysfunctions can offer fellow professionals specific guidance and assistance to supplement the suggestions made here. Eye movements are a fine level of differentiated movement that evolve with developmental control of the body. Direct therapeutic handling permits the system to experience more normal feedback with the assistance of the therapist. This direct experience is the essential cue for the central nervous system to initiate action that will provide feedback within the system itself. As normal responses begin to outnumber the abnormal, a shift in functional balance occurs, and the person changes posture, movement and behavior. Vision as a primary sense and posture as a base for controlled movement must be seen as an interactional system to facilitate optimal change in multihandicapped individuals.

CHAPTER XIII

EVALUATING QUALITY IN MOTOR BEHAVIOR

An appreciation for the complex nature of praxis is essential for the therapist interested in the effective treatment of movement and posture disorder. Praxis in and of itself is man's kinetic vehicle for action. Each sequence of movement must be supported by postural control and a delicate organization of dissociated integration. This dissociation refers to the ability for independent movement of the primary body musculature groups, such as the head and neck, eyes, shoulders, trunk, pelvis, and upper and lower extremities. Organizing this dissociation or independence is the basic process of coordination. It provides man with the ability to apply coordination to activities that require manipulative skill, resulting in meaningful function. Function, therefore, might be described as the integration of dissociated freedom that leads to skilled movement behavior.

Skilled movement behavior has traditionally been the focus of much of the therapeutic intervention strategies surrounding children with physical disabilities. Historically, emphasis has been placed on reflexology, both primitive and pathological, motoric milestones based on averages of developmental maturation in normal children, and manual dexterity as a function of speed and accuracy of manipulation. Application of these evaluations of motor behavior has been successful in identifying the obvious restrictions of physically disabled children or the incoordination of the observably clumsy child. They have provided developmental age levels as a kind of motor IQ, which identifies how far below the child is functioning compared to the motor skill of other children of like chronological age. However, therapists and other students of movement and posture must rely heavily on subjective judgment when it comes to the quality of movement or the degree of coordination in the absence of milestone achievement.

Understanding and identifying quality in motor behavior is dependent on a firm knowledge of the underlying foundations of skilled praxis. These foundations include the proprioceptive and kinesthetic sensory systems, the various components of movement that make up a pattern of motion, and the almost infinite integrative relationships of these dissociated components. To be sure, the creative magic of movement is in its infinite variety, and its magnetic beauty is in the harmonious transition from one position to another. The same movement can have the grace of a ballet or the fierce power of athletic combat. The personality of the movement pattern is as essential to understand as the components of the movement pattern. Movement and posture are man's demonstrative tools of intelligence, emotion, and skill. Almost every behavioral evaluation in some way depends on an intact movement system. If the underlying proprioceptive foundation is not considered in the failure or absence of a tested skill, then the conclusions for failure and indeed its remediation may well be misguided.

Identifying Movement Quality

Developmentally, the newborn demonstrates patterns of movement that have been called reflexive. The important point to consider about newborn movement patterns is the nature of the total body response. The infant moves in total patterns, first asymmetrically as in the well-known tonic neck reactions and then several months later more symmetrically in prone and supine extension and flexion. These total pattern responses serve to develop postural tone to support antigravity control. Once a postural background of tone exists, the child begins to separate out various movements and body parts. This separation or dissociation of body movements is the basis of rotation around the body axis. Rotation is what allows smooth and graded transition from one posture to another. Quality of movement to a large extent is dependent on rotation as an integrator of dissociation. All movement patterns and highly refined skills are essential, varying combinations of flexion extension and rotation. Each pattern biases or activates the others, and each pattern of extension flexion and rotation is made up of movement components of the head, neck, shoulders, trunk, extremities, pelvis, and so on. Each component biases and activates the others. Normal movement requires a harmonious communication of components and patterns.

Abnormal movement or incoordination ia first observed as out of place or unpleasant because there is no harmony, beauty or creativity. The abnormal movement or uncoordinated, clumsy movement is also made up of patterns and component parts. They bias and activate each other just as in normal movement; however, they lack variety and adaptability. Abnormal movement is often characterized as stereotypic or recurring because the child's effort to move or perform a coordinated act results in the same disorganized or abnormal outcome. All abnormal or uncoordinated movement is made up of varying combinations of flexion, extension and rotation. Understanding normal movement components leads directly to an understanding of abnormal components and allows for quality judgments.

There are several guides that can be used to assist the therapist in analyzing quality in movement and posture: starting position, initiation of movement, transition and final position. The starting position determines a great deal in the outcome of control. Movement is initiated with a change in starting position. For example, standing up from a supine position would require a different pattern than standing up from a crawling position. The entire sequence of movements and components is completely different. The combinations of flexion, extension and rotation are completely unrelated in the two different transitions to stand.

The patterns used to stand in the above examples are dependent on underlying factors of starting position. The alignment of the body parts to each other biases what movements are available. The distribution of weight influences and is influenced by alignment and determines which movements are likely to take place first. For instance, lying supine in symmetry would provide an equal distribution of weight, and the possibilities for standing would be unencumbered, whether the movement was initiated symmetrically straight up or rotation was used first to go to prone or side sitting prior to the upright stance. If the starting position happened to be with the head and trunk significantly aligned to one side of the pelvis and legs, it is unlikely that a symmetrical potential for initial movement would be possible. More likely, the initial posturing would be a prop to side sitting and then an organized upright attempt once weight distribution was more advantageous.

Initiation of movement refers to which body part(s) moves first. The initiating part will have direct influence on the component movements that follow in support and cooperation. For example, if the first movement is from the head and neck, then the shoulders and trunk, etc., will follow cooperatively in support of the intent and inertia set in motion. Movement can be initiated from any part of the body. The combinations of flexion, extension and rotation will vary depending on initiation point as well as the degree of importance and support of underlying components of movement. For instance, standing from "four point" by initiating the legs to come into more flexion and placed underneath the trunk for support in standing requires the head to drop or stay steady and the body weight to go forward on the hands. Initiating from the head by elevating to horizontal shifts the weight back over the knees, and the resultant kneel prepares for standing through a half-kneel.

Inability to initiate or disorganized initiation causes a ripple effect that prevents the component movements from cooperating harmoniously and disorganizes or prevents the required interaction of flexion, extension and rotational patterns. It is virtually impossible to stand up from the supine position when the head is kept back against the surface. The rest of the body, struggle as it might, cannot organize a successful attempt at standing. If the head makes the initial move, but the eyes do not correspond with and adjust to the movement, the head posture may be diverted and lead to incoordination in the sequence. If the eyes make the initial movement, but the neck musculature is unable to respond properly, the eyes will be diverted from pursuit, and the movement to visually orient will be abandoned or clumsy. Any problem in initiation or cooperation of other component parts can cause an interruption in the harmony and coordination of movement and posture.

Transition requires that the starting position and initiation is followed by the harmonious cooperation described above. Transition is the equalizer to changes in the center of gravity caused by the inertia of movement. Transition, or rotational force, balances the flexion and extension and corrects the relationship between components and patterns as the distribution of weight is changed from side to side or forward and back. (Although vestibular and non-vestibular proprioceptors are at the foundation for all movement, this discussion will emphasize the actual patterns and components of movement and not the sensory or neurological basis for movement.) Understanding transition means appreciating weight distribution and its effect on the mobility and stability factors of organized movement. Returning to standing from a crawling position, if the weight distribution is not maintained properly, too much weight may be transferred forward, causing a collapse. If not enough weight is transferred forward, the legs will not be able to come under the trunk in an alignment appropriate for a controlled transition to standing.

The final position is the desired new postural alignment, in our example, standing. The final position is essentially a new starting position, and the loop continues from movement to movement and posture to posture. If the final position is compromised in some way, then the starting position for the next movement will compromise the efficiency and coordination of the next sequence and so on into the loop of abnormal, stereotypic or clumsy movements so characteristic of the disabled population.

Developing Criteria for Movement Analysis
Because the nature of movement is so variable and diverse, simple evaluations of developmental milestones do not adequately relate to the infinite variety of ways for a child to demonstrate the milestone. In fact, the way in which a child achieves the ability to hop, skip and jump is unimportant. For every person alive there is a different way to hop, skip and jump. The important factor is in the quality of the success or failure.

If the goal is to hop, how will its success or failure be determined? What will be the criteria? Distance off the ground? Number of hops per minute? If these criteria are not met, then what is the conclusion? Failure? Practice harder? If the goal is to hop, the understanding of the failure to hop requires criteria analysis. For example, does the child's head bend too far forward to the point of losing the starting position? Does the child lift each foot off the surface individually because he cannot shift his weight forward but only side to side? Does the child make one jump or get worse in hopping and at the same time initiate the hop in more and more extension? The list of possible criteria can go on and on, and only those criteria which are appropriate for analysis of a particular movement need to be considered. Using criteria-based referencing to analyze movement can be a valuable tool in targeting underlying movement dysfunction and providing specificity for intervention, as well as a means to evaluate remedial effectiveness.

Introduction to Criteria-Testing

Clinical judgment plays a major role in the use and effectiveness of therapeutic procedures. Observational skill of the therapist is a key determinant to the development and application of treatment. Often the progress of a child is expressed in subjective terminology based on observations of movement and posture of the child under treatment. Evaluating performance based on quality has always been impossible to standardize due to its judgmental nature. Nevertheless, therapists continue to depend on such judgments due to the lack of measurable standards for the infinite variety of performance possibilities, both educationally and developmentally, in the everyday life of the child.

This assessment tool provides a guide to the observation and interpretation of quality analysis of movement and posture parameters necessary for skilled performance. This evaluation can be used for assisting in the clinical observation of motor patterns or can be applied to any specific learning or performance task.

Subtests are designed to assist the therapist in determining and analyzing the normal and abnormal components of movement and posture. Subtests can be used as presented in this evaluation or additional components can be included. Any number of subtests can be developed exclusively by the administering therapist without changing the concept or scoring procedure of the evaluation.

Appropriate use of this tool should allow the therapist to develop increased observational skills and appreciation of the complicated process of motor praxis, target habitual postural fixations or stereotypic movement components, provide more discrete intervention, and document changes in praxis over specific treatment intervals. The criteria-based reference format provides the therapist with the means to identify, analyze and interpret subjective data in a more controlled and precise manner.

Criteria-Based Reference Formatting
The following discussion may be helpful in evaluating the effects of lenses and/or prisms on neuro-motor function.

Criteria-based formatting essentially means that a specific criterion has been established for determination. This can simply be the performance of a skill, such as catching a ball, or a more specific component of that skill, such as raising both arms in preparation for catching. In either case, the goal is not to determine the child's developmental level or standard error of deviation from a mean performance of his peers, but to determine success or failure. The child either caught the ball or he didn't. The child either raised both hands or he didn't.

Criteria-based referencing has value in that it allows the subject to serve as his own control. The subject competes against his own established criteria. Although these criteria are not dependent on developmental skill levels, such levels and the child's maturation need to be considered when developing and interpreting criteria references for any individual task. In addition, developmental levels can be surmised and associated with criteria referencing by associating the child's developmental age with existing standardized performance scales.

Using criteria referencing to assist in analyzing quality movement components requires the therapist to examine the process by which the child performs the task. For example, the fact that a child can catch a ball has relatively little meaning in terms of quality of response. This problem has long been identified as a weakness of developmental milestone testing. If the child, for example, catches the ball by closing his eyes, holding his breath, and clutching the ball to his breast, it can hardly be considered a skilled performance, albeit a successful one. Although therapists make observational notations of such behaviors, there is not always a means to quantify these observations.

Considering the above example, a criteria-referenced attempt to quantify quality observations of performance might result in some of the following criteria-based questions:

1. Does the child stand in normal alignment to begin the task?

2. Does the child keep head aligned to initiate reaching of arms?

3. Do the arms reach bilaterally with extension in parallel?

4. Do the eyes maintain contact with the target?

5. Etc.

If any of the established criteria is answered no, then the therapist must analyze the component parts of that step in the performance. For example, if #2 above is answered, no, then all we know is that the head did not maintain alignment. The significance of this problem must then be determined. Possible questions to help in discovering underlying dysfunction might include the following:

2. Does the head drop with shoulder elevation?

2. Does the head/neck hyperextend with reaching?

159

2. Do the eyes close before head movement?

2. Do the eyes move up or down before head movement?

2. Does the head posture to R or L? (circle one)

2. Does the child flex forward or turn away completely?

2. Etc. (Note that each subpart is #2 to correspond to the original normal criteria.)

The significance of such an investigation can assist the therapist in identifying possible causal relationships. In the above example it may be discovered that the child throws his head back when the ball is tossed. This might be found to be preceded by eye movement upward, resulting in the arms becoming disorganized in reaching. Perhaps the child's dissociation of eye, head and neck is the main cause of the trouble and not the more obvious level of eye-hand coordination. A targeted investigation of the relationship of neck musculature, head and eye movement, visual field orientation, and the like becomes a logical starting point rather than bilateral hand activities or practice sessions at catching a ball.

Using criteria-based reference formatting in the above-described way can be helpful to the therapist in becoming more precise in evaluating underlying causes to performance failures and targeting intervention strategies to the underlying problem. Additionally, such a criteria referencing can assist the therapist in documenting change. For example, the child may have had no success at catching a ball due to the underlying postural disorganization. After establishing better organization for the child, the therapist can evaluate the level of intervention success by readministration. Even if the child can still not catch a ball consistently on a normal level, perhaps the criteria will show a change in head and eye participation. At this point appropriate practice would be in order to give the child experience in organizing the newly established, more normal components, just as learning normally takes place.

SUBTEST #3 (Sample)

Client's Name:

Description: Prone Reach

Starting Position: Person starts in prone after demonstration by therapist of starting position and movement requested.

Instructions: Therapist demonstrates starting position, elbows and arms at 90 degrees, extends arms and legs into a pivot prone position.

Command: "Now you do the same thing. When I say 'Go,' reach up toward my hands and hold for 10 seconds." (Repeat three times.)

	Quality Performance Listing	Attempts 123 123
1.	Does the person start from a symmetrical position in prone?	Yes___No___
2.	Does child lift legs and arms together in extension?	Yes___No___
3.	Do the elbows remain extended in reach?	Yes___No___
4.	Do the hands remain open and relaxed?	Yes___No___
5.	Is the weight distributed primarily on stomach?	Yes___No___
6.	Do the knees remain extended?	Yes___No___
7.	Does the head lift and remain up in alignment with trunk?	Yes___No___

8. Do the shoulders remain relaxed and stable during holding?   Yes___No___

9. Does the person return smoothly to the starting position?   Yes___No___

10.   Yes___No___

11.   Yes___No___

12.   Yes___No___

13.   Yes___No___

14.   Yes___No___

15.   Yes___No___

Score 1 point for each yes answer only.   1 2 3
Total yes points   ___ ___ ___

Problem Performance Listing	Attempts
	123 123
1. Is the person's upper body aligned to the right of the lower body?	Yes___No___
1. Is the person's upper body aligned to the left of lower body?	Yes___No___
1. Is the right leg internally rotated?	Yes___No___
1. Is the left leg internally rotated?	Yes___No___
2. Does the person keep head down or lift with difficulty?	Yes___No___

2. Do the arms remain flexed? Yes___No___

2. Do the shoulders elevate and tighten? Yes___No___

2. Do the legs lift only? Yes___No___

2. Does the upper body lift only? Yes___No___

2. Do legs lift first, then uppers attain desired posture? Yes___No___

2. Does head/trunk lift first, then legs attain posture? Yes___No___

2. Does the person list to the right or left? (Circle R or L.) Yes___No___

3. Do elbows remain flexed? (Circle more on R or L.) Yes___No___

4. Are hands fisted? (Circle more on R or L.) Yes___No___

5. Is weight distribution mostly on trunk with head/arms only up? Yes___No___

5. Is weight distribution on upper legs with only knees bent? Yes___No___

6. Are knees flexed? (Circle more on R or L.) Yes___No___

7. Do head and neck show extreme hyperextension? Yes___No___

7. Does head posture against arm for stability? (Circle R or L.) Yes___No___

8. Do shoulders elevate and tighten to hold in lifting? Yes___No___

9. Does the person collapse from posture after holding? Yes___No___

10. Yes___No___

11. Yes___No___

12. Yes___No___

13. Yes___No___

14. Yes___No___

15. Yes___No___

Score a fraction of 1 point based on the sum of items of like number answered yes. If four #1s are yes, each = 1/4 point, if three #1s are yes, each = 1/3.   1   2   3

    Total yes points   ___ ___ ___

SCORING CHART

Subtest #:

Instructions: Place a check under each body area for each "yes" answer scored under the problem performance listing questions.

```
                       1 2 3
Subtest Max            _____              DISTRIBUTION
Quality Score         -_____              head/neck
                                          _____
Dysfunction Factor    =_____        R.hand/shdr.   L.shdr./hand
                                    _____            _____
Dysfunction % score   =_____  _____      trunk      _____
                                    R._____  _____L.
                                            pelvis
                                    R._____  _____L.
(Place a check mark in each
area of a yes answer on the         R.leg _____  _____L.leg
problem performance listing.)       R.foot_____  _____L.foot
```

INTERPRETATION

MAJOR IMPRESSIONS OF DISTRIBUTION:

Application of Criteria-Based Analysis

Criteria-based reference formatting can be used to evaluate a specific motor task, whether it be in a child with cerebral palsy, a child with incoordination associated with learning disability, or an adult with a traumatic brain injury. The primary requirement in using this format is to fully observe and analyze the task and its component parts, describe behaviorally the normal sequence of events, and then identify possible dysfunctional components within each normal event of the sequence.

This type of analysis can be used to evaluate various intervention techniques. The initial analysis provides a base line for the person's performance. Following intervention, retesting can provide information as to the possible effectiveness of treatment based on documented changes in the component performance of the task. Theoretically, this type of analysis could be used to evaluate visual training influences on movement coordination, the use of prism lenses on movement and posture, the effectiveness of physical intervention in occupational or physical therapy utilizing neurodevelopmental treatment (NDT), or other forms of treatment techniques.

CHAPTER XIV

POST-TRAUMA VISION SYNDROME CAUSED BY HEAD INJURY

Traumatic brain injury (TBI) is devastating to an individual and to the family. Family members and loved ones have great difficulty dealing with the suddenness of the injury, which can result in deep coma or multiple problems with motor function, speech and cognition. Many survivors of traumatic brain injury will have an understanding or recollection of normalcy but will experience bewilderment in their new-found situation. Psychologically, this state can cause severe depression, anger, frustration and a feeling of helplessness.

In traumatic brain injury cases immediate attention is to emergency and medical needs of the victim. The medical team involved in primary treatment will aim their directions at coping with the survival needs of the patient. At the hospital, new teams of physicians and paramedical professionals will continue to address the emergency of the physical trauma. If the individual is in a coma, special medical treatment programs will be initiated.

Decisions will be made quickly by medical teams. Their treatment directions may often require quick decision making by family and loved ones regarding surgical or medical intervention. The immediate family often struggles to understand medical terms and treatment regimens so that appropriate decisions can be made.

Once the individual recovers from the coma, hard realities of physical limitations and cognitive function must be addressed. While medical treatment programs and surgical intervention may still need to be carried out and decisions made to enable continued recovery from the trauma, now the family and medical teams must also deal with the rehabilitation. During this period, family members must cope with the realization that life styles will change and that treatment programs for rehabilitation will continue for long periods of time, if not indefinitely. Many will experience denial, depression, and psychological states that will also need treatment from the appropriate professionals.

As the individual recovers from the coma, testing is done to determine levels of function. The testing may involve metabolic and medical tests as well as electro-physiological tests to determine states of brain function and central nervous system involvement. From these tests physicians, physical therapists, occupational therapists and other professionals will determine appropriate modes of rehabilitation. The team might also include psychologists, cognitive rehabilitation specialists, speech pathologists, neurologists, all of whom will decide on particular forms of therapy necessary to attempt to bring the patient to his maximum potential state of rehabilitation.

The purpose of this brief discussion is to orient the reader to the immediate and long-term directions that are required for the person who has traumatic brain injury. Treatment programs begin with emergency procedures and then slowly blend into the form of medical and physical rehabilitative functions as well as psychological counseling.

If there are any concerns regarding possible ocular problems, an ophthalmologist will be called to join the emergency team early on in the treatment program. The ophthalmological evaluation will attempt to determine if the trauma has caused an impairment to the sight. If no ocular problems exist and the patient is placed into a rehabilitative program, professionals may find that certain aspects of performance do not meet the expectations of the therapist. At that time an eye examination would usually be recommended.

Unfortunately, it has been observed that throughout medical and rehabilitative treatment programs little regard is given to the individual's level of visual function. Even in later stages of rehabilitation, if a question is raised with regard to a visual interference that may be a result of the traumatic brain injury, the examination may be to emphasize needs of sight as opposed to visual function.

The majority of individuals who recover from a traumatic brain injury will have binocular function difficulties in the form of strabismus, oculomotor dysfunction, convergence and accommodative abnormalities. The abruptness of the binocular function problem makes compensation difficult, leading in many cases to horror fusionalis (diplopia or double vision). When a condition such as this occurs, an obstacle or interference exists that causes the individual to have to either compensate or be unable to function in a way that is expected. For a person who has had a traumatic brain injury, compensation for a binocular function problem may be quite difficult. For example, many individuals will have an exotropia as a result of the TBI. When this condition occurs in the normal development of a child, the brain will adapt by suppressing central vision in the strabismic eye. However, when the condition occurs abruptly, as in TBI, the brain will not have had a chance to adapt gradually, and in many cases it is quite possible that the individual is left with horror fusionalis. This condition can severely affect recovery from the TBI. All past experiences were based on an individual visual world. The double vision interferes with depth judgment and object localization, and the ability to match visual information with kinesthetic, proprioceptive and vestibular experiences becomes greatly interrupted. In turn, balance, coordination and movement become affected. Movements will often appear clumsy. Also, fixations, as well as eye movements, may appear to be quite varied.

Unfortunately, for many individuals with a TBI, past experiences that developed when vision and motor processes were intact have little meaning with new levels of motor and cognitive dysfunction. The therapist, in an attempt to provide an appropriate medium for the matching and transferring of past experiences to new situations, will encounter great difficulties when the visual system cannot achieve a balance to enable past experiences to be matched appropriately. Due to the major impact of the visual system on cognitive function and motor development, the visual rehabilitative needs of the TBI patient must be addressed as early as possible and integrated into all aspects of the rehabilitation program.

The insult to the cortex produced from a traumatic brain injury causes stress in the central and autonomic nervous systems. The effect on vision seems to be an interference with the ambient process that primarily affects peripheral fusion and spatial organization. It is postulated that the disruption occurs at the level of midbrain, where vision is matched with kinesthetic, proprioceptive, and vestibular processes. Strabismus may result or a phoria may occur. While exophoria is more common, vertical tropias, esotropia, or esophoria have also been noted. An actual deviation of the eye, with the result of horror fusionalis or diplopia, causes disruption in motor function. It will be observed that the person experiencing this condition will demonstrate limitation to ocular movements as well as high muscle tone, particularly about the head, neck and shoulder areas. Extension of the head and neck is often observed, as is high tone to muscle tissues and other parts of the body. The severe spatial disorientation that occurs from horror fusionalis may cause the varying states of high muscle tone and extension patterns. Suppression in most cases has not developed since the brain has not adapted to the strabismus. Therefore, individuals will develop abnormalities in head posture.

It has been observed that even with extremely low-functioning persons, after traumatic brain injury, head postures will be developed in an attempt to cover or block vision from one eye. This is often an attempt by the person to compensate for the diplopia. Often therapists do not relate these abnormal postures to visual function. Therapy treatment for these abnormal postures sometimes lack result because the treatment is directed at the symptom and not the cause. While patching of one eye or the other may initially relieve the stress on the visual system, the behaviors which have become habitual compensations in some cases may remain for periods of time after the patching has been ceased. Patching should not be the long-term solution. Patching produces a monocular condition that can cause additional stress on the visual and motor systems and lead to difficulties with midline concepts, thus affecting balance and posture. Treatment should emphasize the design of lenses and/or prisms to reduce the stress on the visual system.

The visual condition that results from a head injury has been termed the Post-Trauma Vision Syndrome (PTVS) (see Figure 5). It has been named this to emphasize that the condition is caused by a disruption to the ambient process of vision, and the exotropia or exophoria that often occurs is a result of the greater visual problem.

POST-TRAUMA VISION SYNDROME

Characteristics:
- Exotropia or High Exophoria
- Accommodative Dysfunction
- Convergence Insufficiency
- Low Blink Rate
- Spatial Disorientation
- Poor Fixations and Pursuits
- Unstable Ambient Vision

Symptoms:
- Possible Diplopia
- Objects Appear To Move
- Poor Concentration and Attention
- Staring Behavior
- Poor Visual Memory
- Astenopic Symptoms
- Associated Neuromotor Difficulties
  - Balance
  - Coordination
  - Posture

Figure 5. Common characteristics and symptoms associated with the post-trauma vision syndrome.

For the low-functioning TBI patient, the examiner must use objective means of testing and analyze behavioral changes that relate to the visual and neurmototor processes. Behavioral observations should include the state of muscle tone, particularly in the neck and shoulder areas. For example, spasticity in the temporal-mandibular joint can sometimes be related to stress from the visual process. Upon the introduction of appropriate lenses and/or prisms, a release of motor spasticity can be observed. Therefore, the examiner must take time to observe postures, movements and motor functions in general. When possible, the examiner should invite other therapists and relatives to the examination, since they have had more experience in observing the patterns of function for that individual. Videotaping the patient during the examination is also very helpful. Changes that were not immediately recognizable often become apparent when reviewing the tape.

For TBI patients of higher function who may be able to sit, stand, walk, and respond either motorically and/or verbally, testing should proceed beyond the examination chair. It is very important to observe postural adaptations and compensations while sitting in different seats, walking and also standing. Speech patterns may also be affected by the Post-Trauma Vision Syndrome and a speech therapist may be helpful in determining the effects of lenses and prisms on language and speech function.

When previous prescriptions are available, the examiner should utilize them to determine changes that have resulted from the traumatic brain injury. The examiner must never assume that because an individual had a prescription prior to the TBI that that prescription should remain the same. The Post-Trauma Vision Syndrome is the result of dysfunction and stress in the central and autonomic nervous systems, thus affecting the ambient visual process. This in turn causes imbalanced states of neuromotor function. It is likely that these neuromotor imbalances will also cause imbalances in refractive and accommodative states of function as well as in ocular alignment. The clinician should consider that vision treatment programs for the traumatic brain-injured person affect the neuromotor system and vice versa. When the clinician prescribes lenses for the TBI patient, the emphasis should be to balance the visual system, which will in turn affect neuromotor function. When possible, lens prescriptions should be balanced between the two eyes. Initially, if it is not possible to prescribe equal powers of lenses, prescription changes should be directed toward balancing the prescriptions for the two eyes as the visual system becomes more flexible in adapting the process of vision.

Considering that the visual process plays a primary role in neuromotor organization and cognitive development, it is important that the visual process be examined early in the rehabilitation of persons with traumatic brain injury. The visual system will demonstrate changes that are a direct result of the insult to the cortex. These changes will be in both refractive imbalances and oculomotor states affecting fusional abilities, eye teaming responses, fixation, saccades and other sensory-motor relationships. The earlier visual intervention can be established, the faster and more complete the recovery. Visual intervention should include a behavioral approach to incorporate the important relationships of vision and motor abilities.

When developing a rehabilitation program for vision, the examiner must keep in mind several factors that seem to typify those patients who have had a traumatic brain injury. In a recent study at a hospital for traumatic brain-injured persons, the author chose ten patients for a random sample. The examination of these patients revealed a very high incidence of exotropia and exophoria, the former being an eye deviated outward, the latter indicating a tendency for the eye to align on a point in space further than the object of regard. Traditionally, these conditions are thought of as simply a muscle imbalance of the eyes. However, the visual system is really a relationship of sensory-motor functions throughout the body, and these functions are controlled and organized in the brain. It appears that the insult to the cortex disrupts function of the ambient visual process. The eye alignment imbalance of exophoria or exotropia is a result of this. The exophoria and exotropia that result in a large number of TBI patients may therefore be thought of as a characteristic of the Post-Trauma Vision Syndrome. In other words, the balance of eye alignment indicates the relationship between the ambient visual process and the motor-sensory balances in the body.

In normally sighted patients who have not had traumatic brain injury but have exophoria or exotropia, behavioral observations reveal symptoms of staring, frequent daydreaming, loss of comprehension when reading, having to reread to understand context, a lack of attention and concentration abilities particularly at near vision activities, peripheral distractibility, spatial disorientation and generally poor organization abilities. It is interesting to observe that many of these symptoms become manifested for TBI patients who also have a high amount of exophoria or exotropia. The condition of exophoria is not just a muscle imbalance. It is the barometer of motor and sensory organization status for the individual.

Relating back to the detailed discussion of focal and ambient processing, individuals with a high amount of exophoria that has resulted from a traumatic brain injury will be very ambient in the nature of their visual system. Many patients who can respond verbally will discuss their visual instability. One patient explained that everything he looked at moved and often objects or persons would appear distorted. He described is as:

> ...a world that visually makes no sense. It constantly changes--but I will not be fooled--I know that it cannot be this way even though there is no order to things....

Faces would stretch in different directions, and when he walked, the walls moved and the floor appeared to bend and bow before him. Obviously for this individual, mobility was a very difficult accomplishment. He also had a high muscle tone in his head, neck and shoulder areas which restricted upper body movements.

In treating patients with Post-Trauma Vision Syndrome, it has been found that a low amount of base-in prism can be very effective in reducing stress in the ambient visual process. Two prism diopters base-in before each eye (in addition to distance refractive prescription) can very often reduce and even eliminate many of these bizarre symptoms that are experienced by the patient. The base-in prism reduces peripheral fusion demand on the ambient process, thereby relieving stress on the oculomotor system. In turn, it helps establish a new relationship to the sensory-motor aspect of the visual process, thus affecting spatial and temporal relationships. As the visual stress is relieved primarily in the ambient function of vision, the focal vision process improves in function, thereby affecting the higher perceptual processes; attention and concentration also being affected. The author has found that individuals will respond quickly to the base-in prism prescription, reporting that they feel more comfortable or that their vision seems more stable. In addition, walking patterns and posture can also change.

For the individual discussed in the previous paragraph who had the unstable nature to his visual system, the base-in prism enabled him to walk without experiencing movement in the walls and floor, and he no longer experienced the distortion of his visual world. He explained that the effect of the base-in prism was to enable him to now "understand" his visual world. This statement of understanding the visual world underscores the important but delicate balance of cognitive function as it relates to motor and sensory processing.

This same patient, when attempting to read, would hold his hand up to block off peripheral information from the page. He explained that when he was trying to look at a word on the page, everything else on the page became an extreme distraction, and he had to physically block off all other areas of the page. With the low amount of base-in prism he felt more comfortable as he read, and he had better control over the peripheral areas of his vision.

An explanation for this is that his visual system was highly ambient in function, and that he could not suspend peripheral visual information in order to organize focal vision processing. The base-in prism alone was not enough for developing reading abilities. It was found that patching in the temporal area of reading lenses was very important to help him block off peripheral areas of vision. Blocking peripheral vision enabled him to develop his focal function of the visual process with greater ease. For this patient the base-in prism was also found to relieve a high tonicity of muscle tissue in the neck and shoulder areas. This enabled the physical and occupational therapists to increase the range of motion of the head and neck, as well as to improve fine motor capabilities.

The author recalls that initially when this patient was examined, questions about his visual function had to be directed to his wife because he appeared to be severely confused and disoriented. Since the treatment program has been established with prescriptive lenses and vision therapy, it is interesting to note that the patient now responds directly to the examiner. In a team meeting with his physiatrist, neurologist, therapists and psychologist, significant progress has been reported in cognitive function. The psychologist reported that the patient now has much greater ability to establish time continuity in both speech and motor organizational patterns, and that the patient now has more normal conversational patterns that were not expected from earlier testing.

Not all TBI patients require temporal patching. In some cases nasal patches will be effective in providing structure to their visual field. However, the examiner must be sensitive to the high ambient component of the visual process causing PTVS. For some individuals, if base-in prism is not enough to help him totally control this ambient function, then temporal or nasal patching may assist further in being able to organize peripheral information.

Again, it must be emphasized that the visual system relates to motor function as well as to cognitive organizational abilities. Speech patterns, thought patterns, perceptual abilities are all going to be affected when the visual system, as a processing system, is interrupted. If visual rehabilitation for the TBI patient can be provided in a behavioral way to attempt to re-establish visual organization, then functional capabilities in other areas will also be affected.

For individuals who are very low functioning, prism therapy regimens can be very effective in attempting to re-establish balances in the oculomotor and sensory component of vision. Yoked prisms (the base end of the prism placed in the same orientation for both eyes) can be very effective in making changes in the oculomotor state, which thereby affects sensory function. Each time a prism is introduced before the eyes of an individual in a tandem or yoked fashion as described, the eyes will reorient to look at the image of the object in a new position in space. The prism simply shifts the object to a new position. The muscles of the eyes will turn the eyes to look at the object at this position in space. When the motor system readjusts, it sends information to the cortex, which states that the sensory component must readapt itself to this new position in space. This effect causes a reorientation of motor and sensory organization in the cortex. For example, if an individual were to have base-up prism placed before his eyes, the sensory component of the visual system would see the world much lower than what he had previously experienced. The muscles of the eyes deviate the eyes downward, causing the oculomotor system to relate to the cortex that since the eyes are being turned downward, the environment must be in a lower position. The general orientation to the environment established through the motor component of the eyes causes the individual to change his balance and alignment to gravity. This problem-solving approach through the visual system causes the motor system to lean forward as if the person were walking down a hill.

The opposite effect occurs when base-down is introduced before both eyes. The environment being shifted upward causes the eye muscles to shift upward. Information received by the cortex from the extra-ocular muscles reorients the sensory component of vision as well as the entire motor component in the body. Posture is readjusted so that the person experiences the effect of walking up a hill, thereby reducing flexion. The visual component is so strong that it can cause the individual's relationship to the environment to actually change, and there will be a shift in weight backward as if reorienting to a shift in gravity. This shift in orientation to space may at first seem quite simplistic. One might believe that if the person shifts his weight in one direction or the other as an adaptation to the prism, once the shift is made everything will appear the same. In reality, the effect of making a postural change to space occurs as a problem-solving attempt by the individual to deal with his spatial environment through a vision-neuro-motor relationship. If the person is successful in making this shift in motor orientation, it occurs not simply because of the eye muscles changing in position, but because information is matched and re-established between the sensory component of vision, the motor component of vision, the vestibular process, the kinesthetic and the proprioceptive inputs to the brain. The visual system should act to re-establish the balances between these systems when yoked prisms are utilized. Therefore, yoked prisms are an important approach for rehabilitation of the person.

Bases-left or bases-right prisms can similarly be effective. With lateral yoked prisms there is a spatial change to the left or to the right, depending upon the type of prism used. Wearing yoked bases-left or -right prisms while attempting to walk will produce some interesting motoric changes. Very often posture will change due to the fact that the person will visually experience the environment as being slanted to the left or right, depending upon the type of prism. This orientation to space will cause the person to experience a weight shift to the left or the right because the perception of their midline is shifted. Utilizing a base-left or a base- right prism can be very effective in attempting to orient the person to the left or right side of his body, particularly in cases involving a hemiplagia.

For individuals who have had a traumatic brain injury and suffer from PTVS, there will very often be weakness on the left or right side of the body that causes him to place more of his weight to one side or the other while sitting, standing, or walking. The concept of midline often is shifted to the opposite, stronger side of his body. Utilizing base-left or base-right prism can reorient the midline through the visual process, thereby causing him to shift his weight to the neglected side of his body.

One patient had a right-side weakness and walked with a cane held in his left hand. The person placed most of his weight on his left foot and developed a limping pattern when weight was placed on his right foot. A test was developed to determine where the individual perceived his own midline. The examiner stood before the patient and asked him to turn his head until he thought that it was straight. The patient was then asked to look at the small object that the examiner held and to say when the object was directly between his eyes. The examiner proceeded to move an object laterally across the field from left to right. The patient said "Stop" when he thought the object was directly in front of his nose or between his two eyes. The patient moved his eyes in a pursuit fashion laterally across the field. This patient repeatedly told the examiner that the object was directly in front of his nose when in fact it was directly in front of his left eye. When base-left prism (10 prism diopters) was introduced before both eyes and the test was repeated, the patient responded when the object was directly in front of his nose. When the patient walked with this base-left prism, the examiner noted that there was a more equal shift in weight between left and right sides, and that the length of stride increased almost twofold. In addition, the speed of walking also increased. The patient responded that he felt more stable, more comfortable, and began to take longer periods of time without walking with the cane.

Optometrists and ophthalmologists working in this area should not make decisions with regard to elimination of canes or other means of support by themselves. Whenever possible, it is a good idea to work very closely with physical and occupational therapists, preferably those trained in neurodevelopmental treatment. In this particular situation the therapist noted that with the base-left prism the patient demonstrated a shifting of weight in the pelvic area that was previously quite restricted. At the therapist's recommendation, less cane support was necessary while the person continued to use the prisms.

If a clinician is considering the prescription of yoked prisms for a traumatic brain-injured person, an extensive behavioral evaluation with lenses and prisms should be developed. There are several guidelines to follow in the prescription of these lenses. For the higher-functioning TBI patient, evaluate the patient's posture in a seated position. Watch for head turns to the left or right or extension or flexion patterns of the head or neck. Also, examine motor function while walking. Watch for head positional changes that occur only during walking. In addition, observe general alignment of the neck and shoulders in relation to movement of the pelvis when the left and right foot is extended forward. If there is a marked head turn to the left or to the right, the examiner should begin by placing the prism in the base direction of the head turn. For example, if the head turn is toward the right shoulder, base orientation of the prism should be to the right. With the prism in place, varying amounts of prism may be tried, starting at 2 or 4 prism diopters. The amount of power may be increased up to 12 prism or 1.5 prism diopters base right. Fresnel prisms may be effective for trial purposes and for prescription. These are plastic press-on prisms that can be used in varying amounts up to 20 prism diopters. With the prism in place, observe if the head realigns its position and the subsequent affect on posture and movement.

Behavioral testing may be developed as described earlier by moving an object approximately 16 inches from the person's face from left to right or right to left and asking the person to respond when the object is directly in front of his nose or between his eyes. This will help the examiner understand shifts in midline. If head orientation changes and becomes more realigned with the base-left or -right prism, the examiner should also observe other movements with these prisms to determine whether reach may be more accurate, if walking patterns are balanced, and if there is improved weight transfer from left to right sides.

For individuals who are showing a left- or right-side weakness, similar observations should be developed concerning posture in a seated position, reaching, and/or walking. Base-left or -right yoked prisms should be used in an attempt to re-establish midline concepts. When prescribing yoked prisms, the examiner may want to recommend that the prism be used for two-to-three-hour intervals during the day. This doesn't allow total adaptation to the prism and will cause the individual to have to reorganize sensory and motor functions when the prism is not in place.

A lens or prism is an extremely potent means for re-establishing the motor relationships to sensory processes, as well as matching information between vestibular, proprioceptive and kinesthetic stimuli. If the prisms are utilized for several hours at a time, then taken away, very often carry-over will be observed and experienced by the individual after the prisms are removed. The examiner should perform frequent evaluations so that progress may be monitored. Additional types of prisms and/or lenses may be recommended as deemed appropriate for the rehabilitative needs of the patient.

Interestingly, for some individuals, particularly elderly persons who have suffered strokes and long-term TBI patients, the opposite type of prism may often show improved results. For example, a paradoxical effect can occur, causing the midline to shift toward the weaker or neglected side. It appears that long- term compensation to the neuromotor imbalances produces visual distortions causing the room to tilt down toward the impaired side of the person. This may or may not be reported by the person, depending upon his state of cognitive-visual awareness. In this paradoxical case the base of the yoked prism should be placed opposite his impaired side (i.e., if there is a left hemiplegia, place the prism in the base right orientation). This will cause the room to appear more level, thereby affecting weight shift and posture.

Yoked bases-up or bases-down prisms can be used similarly to shift the person's orientation to space. For individuals who have demonstrated extension or flexion patterns, bases-up or bases-down prisms may be effective for changing some of these motor postures. If a TBI patient shows extension and motor spasticity when attempting to walk, very often he will also demonstrate a wide stance and rigid posture. Bases-up prisms can sometimes be effective in enabling the person to experience weight shifts forward. Bases-up prisms have the effect of lowering the visual world, causing the patient to experience the effect of walking down a hill. Sometimes the use of this prism can be effective in causing the person to shift his weight more to the front of his feet as opposed to walking with his weight placed on the heels of his feet. If the clinician can utilize prisms to enable the person to problem-solve by shifting weight, then a major step has been established in rehabilitation, and the patient then begins to establish more control over his environment, posture, movement and orientation to space. With bases-up prisms, if the person experiences a weight shift forward, then it is an experience that will be utilized for future balance relationships. The experience may not change or alter all functions immediately but can be an experience that will enable him variation in function and performance for future demands.

Bases-down prisms can be utilized for individuals who are showing flexion. For one non-ambulatory and wheel-chair-bound individual, flexion of the head and neck was observed, and the person only lifted his head for very short periods of time. The prescription of base-down prism demonstrated an immediate effect, causing the person to lift and reorient his head in line with his torso. Capital flexion was increased. (Capital flexion is the extension of the back of the neck and the decrease in the angle between the chin and the chest. This can only be accomplished when the person lifts his head and orients it in an erect fashion over the spinal column.) Similar affects using lateral yoked prisms have been found when treating wheelchair-bound patients who demonstrate a leaning to the left or the right.

For very low functioning TBI patients the examiner has found that the use of base-in prism and also yoked prisms (bases-up, bases-down, bases-left or bases-right) can be very effective in attempting to re-establish visual sensory-motor function. For the low-functioning patient who is confined to bed or can be moved to a seated position, lenses and prisms may be the only approach to actively establish relationships between motor and sensory processes. The lenses and prisms must be thought of as a potent means of challenging the plasticity of the visual process in relationship to sensory-motor processes. A lens or prism is not just another piece of glass or plastic that corrects visual acuity. The lens or prism can be utilized to establish balances and relationships between sensory-motor and also cognitive functions.

It has been observed that the introduction of base-in, base-up, base-down or base-left prisms may promote a number of visual changes such as increased pursuit activity, increased saccades, changes in blink, relationships, and release of motor spasticity. It has also been interesting to observe some low-functioning TBI patients with extension of the head, neck and jaw. Several minutes after a base-in prism is introduced, there is a release in the extension of the temporal-mandibular joint. When this occurs, patients frequently begin to close their mouths and also masticate, demonstrating spontaneous increased tongue activity. When this was observed by the speech pathologists and other therapists, these professionals found the changes in the temporal-mandibular joint quite significant. In the case of several individuals, this release of extension was found each time the base-in prism was introduced. Often individuals demonstrating extreme extension in the temporal-mandibular joint and in the neck area also show spasticity of the arms and high amounts of exotropia.

Regarding the treatment of strabismus and phorias, it has been the author's experience that it is not necessary to prescribe high amounts of base-in prism to correct for exotropia or exophoria. Many traumatic brain-injured patients will actually show avoidance of high amounts of base-in prism. The examiner should approach the prescription of prism in a conservative manner, starting with low amounts and increasing the prism to the point where positive changes begin to result. As a general rule, only two prism diopters before each eye is necessary for the majority of patients.

The behavioral examination of the traumatic brain-injured patient, particularly the low-functioning patient, may have to be averaged over a series of examinations. This means that if at all possible the examiner should see the patient over several days. When therapists are available, the examiner may recommend the use of special prisms to be used over the course of the examination period with detailed notes made with regard to motor capabilities or other functions so that the therapists can report back to the clinician. The result will be a more detailed understanding of the effects of lenses and prisms and how behaviors may be changed.

Vision therapy can also be developed for the TBI patient suffering from Post-Trauma Vision Syndrome. Dramatic changes in performance have been observed with the utilization of various types of lenses and prisms in repeated weekly therapy sessions, particularly with higher-functioning TBI patients. For the first patient discussed in this chapter, who expressed extreme spatial distortion and disorientation in his visual environment, the examiner provided weekly visual therapy sessions. The vision therapy utilized many different lenses and prism combinations and a variety of perceptual motor activities, including general walking and orientation, reaching, touching and movement activities.

Generally, vision therapy in most optometric offices is developed through specific activities. It is not necessarily the activity that makes the change for the patient, whether the patient is traumatically brain injured or not. Rather, it is the lens or prism that establishes the change in the visual-motor relationship. Therefore, if therapy is developed for TBI patients, the procedural activity is not as important as the lenses or prisms that the patient wears during that activity. The most effective vision therapy treatment program is simply to utilize varying types of yoked prisms and enable the person time to experience each through active involvement of the motor system. Initially, for patients who are extremely disoriented in their visual systems, very low amounts of plus lenses in addition to low amounts of yoked prisms should be used, and the amount of prism increased as adaptability is observed.

It is not the intent to develop the area of vision therapy for the TBI in this book. Rather, the emphasis is to establish an understanding of the importance of the visual system to motor function and, further, that through the visual system, motor and cognitive functions can be improved and enhanced. Communication and discussion between professionals involved in occupational, physical, and other modes of therapy, together with the optometric and ophthalmological community regarding this mode of treatment, is the key to change. Optometrists and ophthalmologists need to begin a more behavioral mode of analysis for TBI patients and work with yoked prisms with therapists present so that the therapist's understanding of the motor function can benefit the optometrists and ophthalmologists.

Post-Trauma Vision Syndrome is often a primary interference in rehabilitation after a head injury. Persons with this condition require an aggressive behavioral vision approach to at first reduce stress in the ambient visual process and, second, to re- establish basic visual skills necessary for complete rehabilitation. PTVS is treatable, and the results of treatment emphasize that vision affects neuro-motor function as well as cognitive abilities.

BIBLIOGRAPHY

Albano, ML, B Cox, J York & R York
1981 Educational teams for students with severe and multiple handicaps. R. York, WK Schoefield, DJ Donder, DL Ryndak & B Regnly (Eds.), Organizing and implementing services for students with severe and multiple handicaps. Springfield, IL: Illinois State Board of Education.

Allen, A & P Clark
1985 Occupational therapy for children. St. Louis, MO: C. V. Mosby Company.

Andrezejewska, W & G Baranowska
1969 Accommodation disorders after head injuries and cerebral concussion. Klin Oczna (Poland), July 39 (3):431-5.

Apell, R.
1955 Behavior characteristics of nursery school children. Optom Wkly, Dec 1.

Apell, R & R Lowry
1959 Preschool vision. St. Louis, MO: Am Optom Assoc.

Aracil, P & M Worllez
1985 Usefulness of prisms in paralysis of the superior oblique. Bull Soc Belge Ophthalmol (France) 85 (1):57-9.

Arden, GD
1968 Importance of measuring contrast sensitivity in visual impairment. Br J Ophthalmol: 62.

Ayres, AJ
1973 Sensory integration and learning disorders. Los Angeles, CA: Western Psychological Services.

1979 Sensory integration and the child. Los Angeles, CA: Western Psychological Services.

Back-y-Rita, P.
1980 Recovery of function: theoretical considerations for brain injury rehabilitation. Bern, Switzerland: Hans Heiber Publishers.

Banus, B, M Becker, C Kent, Y Norton & D Sukiennicki
1979 Developmental therapist. Thorofare, NJ: Charles B. Slack, Inc.

Barraga, N.
1965 Effects of experimental teaching on the visual behavior of children with low vision. Am J Optom Arch Am Acad Optom. 42 (9):557-61.

1969 Learning efficiency in low vision. J Am Optom Assoc, 40 (8):807-10.

1979 Development of efficiency in visual functioning: rationale for a comprehensive program. J Vis Impair Blind, 73 (4):93-96.

Bergen, A & C Colangelo
1983 Positioning the client with central nervous system deficits: the wheelchair and other adapted equipment. Valhalla, NY: Valhalla Rehabilitation Publications.

Bernstein, G.
1979 Integration of vision stimulation in the classroom: Part I - individual programming. Education of the Visually Handicapped, 11 (1):14-18.

1979 Integration of vision stimulation in the classroom: Part II - group programming. Education of the Visually Handicapped, 11 (2):39-48.

1979 Integration of vision stimulation in the classroom: Part III - A total approach. Education of the Visually Handicapped, 11 (3):80-84.

Bobath, K.
1959 The neuro pathology of cerebral palsy and its importance in treatment and diagnosis. Cerebral Palsy Bulletin, Vol. 1, No. 8:13-33.

1964 The facilitation of normal postural reactions and movements in the treatment of cerebral palsy. Physiotherapy;, August:3-15.

Borish, I.
1970 Clinical refraction. The Professional Press, Ind.

Brown, L, J Nietupski & S Hamre-Nietupski
1976 The criterion of ultimate functioning and public school services for severely handicapped students. Papers and programs related to public school services for secondary age severely handicapped students, Vol. VI, Part I, Madison Metropolitan School District.

Buktenica, N.
1968 Visual learning. Sioux Falls, SD: Adapt Press, Inc.

Butler, C, T McKay & G Okamota
1985 Mobility cannot wait--powered mobility for very young disabled children. Article obtained while awaiting print in J Devel Med Child Neurology.

Campbell, FW
1974 Contrast and spatial frequency. Sci Am:221.

Campbell, P.
1982 Lecture notes from NDT teacher certification course. Kent State University, Kent, Ohio.

1982 Introduction to neurodevelopmental treatment. Akron, Ohio: Children's Hospital Medical Center, October.

1984 Lecture notes on neurodevelopmental treatment program given at varying sites in Nebraska, April.

Carroll, R & JR Seaber
1974 Acute loss of fusional convergence following head trauma. Am Orthop J, 24:57-59.

Cech, D.
1977 Combining specialities to serve low functioning visually and physically impaired children. J Vis Impair Blind, 71 (10):439- 40.

Cohen, A.
1983 An optometric approach to treatment of non-comitant deviation. J Am Optom Assn, Vol. 54, No. 3, March.

Nebraska State Department of Education
1978 Conference Proceedings from Nebraska Statewide Conference. The deaf/blind/severely/profoundly handicapped.

Corbin, CB.
1980 A textbook of motor development. Dubuque, Iowa: Wm. C. Brown Co. Publishers.

Corn, A.
1981 Optical aids in the classroom. Education for the Visually Handicapped, 12 (4):114-121.

Cullen, C.
1986 Contoured components on adaptive seating devices. Clin Management Phys Therapy, Vol. 6, No. 5:12-13.

Dartmouth Medical School
1974 A study and development of optical devices to aid persons with subnormal vision: a final report to the national research council, committee on sensory devices. Hanover, New Hampshire, Eye Institute.

Faye, EE.
1965 Management of the low vision patient. Int Ophthalmol, 5:495. Faye, EE.

1975 Low vision services in an agency. New Outlook, 4:241-248.
1984 Clinical low vision. Little-Brown, Inc.

Finnie, N.
1975 Handling the young cerebral palsy child at home. New York: E. P. Dutton.

Forrest, E.
1988 Stress and Vision. Optom Extension Prog.

Genensky, S.
1976 Acuity measurements--do they indicate how well a partially sighted person functions or could function? New Outlook (January).

Genensky, S.
1978 Data concerning the partially sighted and functionally blind. J Vis Impair Blind, 72 (5):177-180.

Gesell, A.
1949 Vision, its development in infant and child. New York: Harper and Rowe.

Gesell, A & C Armatruda
1949 Developmental diagnosis. New York: P. B. Hoeber, Inc.

Gianutsos, R & P Matheson
1986 The rehabilitation of visual perceptual disorders attributable to brain injury. Neurological Rehabilitation. M Meier, A Benton, L Diller, Eds. Londen, Churchill Livingston: 202

Gianutsos, R, G Ramsey & R Perlin
1987 Enabling the survivors of brain injury to receive optometric services. J Vis Rehabil.

Gidoni, E & A Milani-Comparetti
1967 Routine developmental examination in normal and retarded children. Developmental Medicine and Child Neurology:631-38.

Gilbert, J.
(1986) The psychological implications of severe visual impairment in older persons. Proceedings on the research conference on geriatric blindness and severe visual impairment. New York: American Foundation for the Blind:43-45.

Gilfoyle, E, A Grady & J Moore
1981 Children adapt. Thorofare, NJ: Charles B. Slack, Inc.

Gnade, M.
1965 Low vision services. Sight-Saving Rev. 35:216.

Hart, CT.
1969 Disturbances of fusion following head injury. Section of Ophthalmology, Vol. 62, July:704-06.

Hatfield, EM.
1973 Estimates of blindness in the United States. Sight-Saving Rev. 43:69-80.

Held, R.
1965 Plasticity in sensory-motor systems. Sci Am, 213 (5):84-95.

Ilg, F & L Ames
1955 Child behavior. New York: Harper and Rowe.

Jose, R, J Cumming & L McAdams
1975 A model of low vision clinical service: an interdisciplinary vision rehabilitation program. New Outlook, 5:249-54.

Jose, R, A Smith & KI Shane
1980 Evaluating and stimulating vision in multiply-impaired. J Vis Impair Blind, 74 (1):2-8.

Jose, R.
1983 Understanding low vision. New York: Am Foundation for Blind.

Kalish, R & S Pressler
1980 Physical and occupational therapy. J School Health (May):264-67.

Kirchner, C & C Lowman
1978 Services of variation in estimated prevalence of visual loss. J Vis Impair Blind 72 (8):329-32.

Kirchner, C & R Peterson
1979 The latest data on visual disability from NCHS. J Vis Impair Blind 73 (4):151-53.

Kirchner, C & R Peterson
1980 Prevalence of blindness and visual impairment among institutional residents. J Vis Impair Blind 74 (8):323-26.

Kirchner, C & B Phillips
1980 Report of a survey of U.S. low vision services. J Vis Impair Blind 74 (3):122-24.

Komph, D, B Neundorfer, W Ehret & CW Wallesch
1977 Transitory impairment of vision after light head trauma in childhood. Neuro-pediatric, Vol. 8, No. 4:354-59.

Krobel, G, R Kristan, J Simon & N Barrows
1986 Post-traumatic convergence insufficiency. Am Ophthalmol, 18 (3) (March):101-2.

Langley, B & R Dubrose
1976 Functional vision screening for severely handicapped children. New Outlook for Blind, 70 (8):346-50.

Langley, B.
1986 Conference notes from SE Region annual meeting of neurodevelopment treatment association. Knoxville, TN, March 14- 16.

Leibowitz, HW & RB Post
1982 The two modes of processing concept and some implications. JJ Beck (Ed) in Organization and Representation in Perception: Hillsdale, NJ, Erlbaum (in press).

Londen, R.
1987 Mono-vision correction for diplopia. J Am Optom Assoc, Vol. 58, No. 7 (July):568.

Lowman, C & C Kirchner
1979 Elderly blind and visually impaired persons: projected numbers in the year 2000. J Vis Impair Blind, 73 (2):73-74.

Lowrey, A.
1965 Plan for a low vision clinic. New Outlook for Blind, 59 (8):275-77.

Meir, M, A Benton & L Diller
1987 Cognitive theories of attention and rehabilitation of attentional deficits. New York, Neuropsychological Rehabilitation:183-201.

National Center for Health Statistics
1971 Prevalence of selected impairments: U.S. Vital and Health Statistics, Series 10, No. 111, DHEW, Pub. No. 77-1537, Washington, DC.

Neisser, U.
1964 Visual search. Sci Amer, 210:94-102.

Padula, WV.
1978 Vision and its influence on development of the visually impaired child. Low Vision Abstracts, Vol. IV, No. 1:1-4.

1979 Philosophy, definition and a model of low vision services. New York: Am Foundation for Blind (Unpublished).

1980 Low vision services. New York: Am Foundation for Blind.

1981 Learning through sensory-motor awareness for the visually impaired person. Presented at American Association for the Blind Conference, Toronto, Canada (Unpublished).

Padula, WV. (R Sekuler, D Kline & K Dismukes, Eds.)
1982 Low vision related to function and service delivery for the elderly. New York: Aging and human visual function, Vol. II, Alan R. Liss Inc.:315-22.

Padula, WV & S Spungin
1982 The visually handicapped child - Part I. The Bridge, Beecher House, Inc.:20-22.

1982 The visually handicapped child - Part II. The Bridge, Beecher House, Inc.:16-18.

Padula, WV & A Dinsmore
1983 Federal low vision services reimbursement, mechanisms. J Am Optom Assoc, Vol. 54, No. 10 (Oct):901-03.

Peterson, D.
1981 Support services. (B Wilcox & R York, Eds.) Quality educational programming for the severely handicapped: the Federal Investment, Washington, DC: Office of Special Education and Rehabilitation Services.

Richter, E.
1982 Sensorimotor assessment and programming (Workshop Notes), sponsored by Nebraska Occupational Therapy Association and Nebraska Chapter of American Physical Therapy Association, Lincoln, NE (May).

Riesen, A.
1947 The development of visual perception in man and chimpanzee. Science 106:107-08.

Rock, I.
1967 Vision and touch. Sci Am, 216 (5):96-104

Smith, E.
1974 Influence of site of impact on cognitive impairment persisting long after severe closed head injury. J Neurol Neurosurgery & Psychiatry, 37:719-26.

Soden, R & AH Cohen
1983 An optometric approach to the treatment of a non-comitant deviation. J Am Optom Assoc, Vol. 54, No. 5 (May):451-54.

Stanworth, A.
1974 Defects of ocular movement and fusion after head injury. Br J ophthalmol, No. 58:266-71.

Stephens, B.
1972 Cognitive processes in the visually impaired. Education of the Visually Handicapped, 4:106-11.

Streff, J.
1976 Gesell Institute of Child Development, Vision Symposium, June

1977 The Cheshire study: changes in incidence of myopia following program of intervention. Frontiers in Visual Science, Springer-Verlag, New York.

Trevarthen, CB & R Sperry
1973 Perceptual unity of the ambient visual field in human commissurotomy patients. Brain, 96:547-70.

Trobe, JR & RM Bauer
1968 Seeing but not recognizing. Survey of Ophthalmology, Vol. 30, No. 5 (March-April):328-36.

Trovern-Trend
1968 Blindness in the United States: A review of the available satistics with estimates of the prevalence of blindness and its economic impact. Hartford, CT: Travelers Research Center.

Warren, D.
1977 Blindness and early childhood development. New York:A'm Foundation for the Blind, Inc.

1982 Workshop notes from "Utilizing adaptive equipment with the school-aged handicapped child. Lincoln, NE, August 27-28.